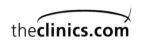

OBSTETRICS AND GYNECOLOGY CLINICS

OF NORTH AMERICA

Teaching and Evaluating Surgical Skills

GUEST EDITOR
Rebecca G. Rogers, MD

CONSULTING EDITOR
William F. Rayburn, MD

June 2006 • Volume 33 • Number 2

SAUNDERS

An Imprint of Elsevier, Inc.
PHILADELPHIA   LONDON   TORONTO   MONTREAL   SYDNEY   TOKYO

W.B. SAUNDERS COMPANY
A Division of Elsevier Inc.

Elsevier, Inc. • 1600 John F. Kennedy Blvd. • Suite 1800 • Philadelphia, PA 19103-2899

http://www.theclinics.com

OBSTETRICS AND GYNECOLOGY
CLINICS OF NORTH AMERICA   Volume 33, Number 2
June 2006   ISSN 0889-8545
Editor: Carla Holloway   ISBN 1-4160-3537-0

Reprints. For copies of 100 or more of articles in this publication, please contact the Commercial Reprints Department, Elsevier Inc., 360 Park Avenue South, New York, New York 10010-1710. Tel.: (212) 633-3818, Fax: (212) 462-1935, email: reprints@elsevier.com

The ideas and opinions expressed in *Obstetrics and Gynecology Clinics of North America* do not necessarily reflect those of the Publisher. The Publisher does not assume any responsibility for any injury and/or damage to persons or property arising out of or related to any use of the material contained in this periodical. The reader is advised to check the appropriate medical literature and the product information currently provided by the manufacturer of each drug to be administered to verify the dosage, the method and duration of administration, or contraindications. It is the responsibility of the treating physician or other health care professional, relying on independent experience and knowledge of the patient, to determine drug dosages and the best treatment for the patient. Mention of any product in this issue should not be construed as endorsement by the contributors, editors, or the Publisher of the product or manufacturers' claims.

Obstetrics and Gynecology Clinics of North America (ISSN 0889-8545) is published quarterly by W.B. Saunders, 360 Park Avenue South, New York, NY 10010-1710. Months of publication are March, June, September, and December. Business and Editorial Offices: 1600 John F. Kennedy Blvd., Suite 1800, Philadelphia, PA 19103-2899. Accounting and Circulation Offices: 6277 Sea Harbor Drive, Orlando, FL 32887-4800. Periodicals postage paid at New York, NY, and additional mailing offices. Subscription prices are $180.00 per year for US individuals, $300.00 per year for US institutions, $90.00 per year for US students and residents, $215.00 per year for Canadian individuals, $370.00 per year for Canadian institutions, $245.00 per year for international individuals, $370.00 per year for international institutions and $125.00 per year for Canadian and foreign students/residents. To receive student/resident rate, orders must be accompanied by name of affiliated institution, date of term, and the signature of program/residency coordinator on institution letterhead. Orders will be billed at individual rate until proof of status is received. Foreign air speed delivery is included in all Clinics subscription prices. All prices are subject to change without notice. POSTMASTER: Send address changes to *Obstetrics and Gynecology Clinics of North America*, Elsevier Periodicals Customer Service, 6277 Sea Harbor Drive, Orlando, FL 32887-4800. **Customer Service: 1-800-654-2452 (US). From outside of the US, call 1-407-345-4000.**

Obstetrics and Gynecology Clinics of North America is also published in Spanish by Mc Graw-Hill Interamericana Editores S.A., P.O. Box 5-237, 06500, Mexico; in Portuguese by Reichmann and Affonso Editores, Rio de Janeiro, Brazil; and in Greek by Paschalidis Medical Publications, Athens, Greece.

Obstetrics and Gynecology Clinics of North America is covered in *Index Medicus, Excerpta Medica, Current Concepts/Clinical Medicine, Science Citation Index, BIOSIS, CINAHL, and ISI/BIOMED.*

Printed in the United States of America.

GOAL STATEMENT

The goal of *Obstetrics and Gynecology Clinics of North America* is to keep practicing physicians up to date with current clinical practice in OB/GYN by providing timely articles reviewing the state of the art in patient care.

ACCREDITATION

The *Obstetrics and Gynecology Clinics of North America* is planned and implemented in accordance with the Essential Areas and Policies of the Accreditation Council for Continuing Medical Education (ACCME) through the joint sponsorship of the University of Virginia School of Medicine and Elsevier. The University of Virginia School of Medicine is accredited by the ACCME to provide continuing medical education for physicians.

NEW The University of Virginia School of Medicine designates this educational activity for a maximum of 15 AMA PRA Category 1 Credits™. Physicians should only claim credit commensurate with the extent of their participation in the activity.

The American Medical Association has determined that physicians not licensed in the US who participate in this CME activity are eligible for 15 AMA PRA Category 1 Credits™.

Category 1 credit can be earned by reading the text material, taking the CME examination online at http://www.theclinics.com/home/cme, and completing the evaluation. After taking the test, you will be required to review any and all incorrect answers. Following completion of the test and evaluation, your credit will be awarded and you may print your certificate.

FACULTY DISCLOSURE/CONFLICT OF INTEREST

The University of Virginia School of Medicine, as an ACCME accredited provider, endorses and strives to comply with the Accreditation Council for Continuing Medical Education (ACCME) Standards of Commercial Support, Commonwealth of Virginia statutes, University of Virginia policies and procedures, and associated federal and private regulations and guidelines on the need for disclosure and monitoring of proprietary and financial interests that may affect the scientific integrity and balance of content delivered in continuing medical education activities under our auspices.

The University of Virginia School of Medicine requires that all CME activities accredited through this institution be developed independently and be scientifically rigorous, balanced and objective in the presentation/discussion of its content, theories and practices.

All authors/editors participating in an accredited CME activity are expected to disclose to the readers relevant financial relationships with commercial entities occurring within the past 12 months (such as grants or research support, employee, consultant, stock holder, member of speakers bureau, etc.). The University of Virginia School of Medicine will employ appropriate mechanisms to resolve potential conflicts of interest to maintain the standards of fair and balanced education to the reader. Questions about specific strategies can be directed to the Office of Continuing Medical Education, University of Virginia School of Medicine, Charlottesville, Virginia.

The authors/editors listed below have identified no professional or financial affiliations for themselves or their spouse/partner:
Dee E. Fenner, MD; Rebecca Hall, PhD; Victoria Handa, MD; Thomas M. Julian, MD; Charles W. Nager, MD; William F. Rayburn, MD, Consulting Editor; Robert A. Starr, MD; Carmen Sultana, MD; Nathan Wagstaff, MD; Andrew J. Walter, MD, FACOOG; and Patrick J. Woodman, DO, FACOOG.

The author listed below identified the following professional or financial affiliations for himself, his spouse/partner:
Kimberly Kenton, MD has institutional grants with Pfizer and Astellas and is conducting clinical trials with Allergan and Q-Med.
Tony Ogburn, MD conducted a research project using IUDs supplied by FEI Women's Health.
Robert M. Rogers, Jr., MD is a consultant and is on the speaker's bureau for Ethicon Women's Health and Urology.

Disclosure of Discussion of non-FDA approved uses for pharmaceutical products and/or medical devices:
The University of Virginia School of Medicine, as an ACCME provider, requires that all faculty presenters identify and disclose any "off label" uses for pharmaceutical and medical device products. The University of Virginia School of Medicine recommends that each physician fully review all the available data on new products or procedures prior to instituting them with patients.

TO ENROLL

To enroll in the *Obstetrics and Gynecology Clinics of North America* Continuing Medical Education program, call customer service at 1-800-654-2452 or visit us online at www.theclinics.com/home/cme. The CME program is available to subscribers for an additional fee of $195.00

CONSULTING EDITOR

WILLIAM F. RAYBURN, MD, Seligman Professor and Chair, Department of Obstetrics and Gynecology, University of New Mexico Health Science Center, Albuquerque, New Mexico

GUEST EDITOR

REBECCA G. ROGERS, MD, Chair, Education Committee, American Urogynecological Society; Director, Division of Urogynecology, Department of Obstetrics and Gynecology, University of New Mexico Health Sciences Center, Albuquerque, New Mexico

CONTRIBUTORS

BETTY CHOU, MD, Department of Gynecology and Obstetrics, Johns Hopkins University School of Medicine, Baltimore, Maryland

DEE E. FENNER, MD, Furlong Professor of Women's Health; Division Head of Gynecology, Department of Obstetrics and Gynecology, University of Michigan Hospital, Ann Arbor, Michigan

REBECCA HALL, PhD, Associate Professor and Clinical Director of Resident/Fellow Ultrasound Program, Department of Obstetrics and Gynecology, University of New Mexico Health Sciences Center, Albuquerque, New Mexico

VICTORIA L. HANDA, MD, Department of Gynecology and Obstetrics, Johns Hopkins University School of Medicine, Baltimore, Maryland

THOMAS M. JULIAN, MD, Professor, Department of Obstetrics and Gynecology, University of Wisconsin Medical School, Madison, Wisconsin

KIMBERLY KENTON, MD, MS, Division of Female Pelvic Medicine and Reconstructive Surgery, Departments of Obstetrics and Gynecology and Urology, Loyola University Medical Center, Maywood, Illinois

CHARLES W. NAGER, MD, Professor of Clinical Reproductive Medicine and Director, Division of Urogynecology, Department of Reproductive Medicine, University of California–San Diego Medical Center, San Diego, California

TONY OGBURN, MD, Associate Professor and Resident Program Director, Department of Obstetrics and Gynecology, University of New Mexico Health Sciences Center, Albuquerque, New Mexico

REBECCA G. ROGERS, MD, Chair, Education Committee, American Urogynecological Society; Director, Division of Urogynecology, Department of Obstetrics and Gynecology, University of New Mexico Health Sciences Center, Albuquerque, New Mexico

ROBERT M. ROGERS, Jr, MD, Northwest Women's Health Center, Kalispell, Montana

ROBERT A. STARR, MD, Director, Divisions of Urogynecology and Gynecology, Department of Obstetrics and Gynecology, William Beaumont Hospital, Royal Oak, Michigan

CARMEN J. SULTANA, MD, Associate Professor, Department of Obstetrics and Gynecology, Jefferson Medical College, Philadelphia, Pennsylvania

NATHAN V. WAGSTAFF, MD, Senior House Officer, Department of Obstetrics and Gynecology, William Beaumont Hospital, Royal Oak, Michigan

ANDREW J. WALTER, MD, Division of Urogynecology, TPMG–Sacramento, Sacramento, California

PATRICK J. WOODMAN, DO, Voluntary Clinical Assistant Professor of Obstetrics and Gynecology, Indiana University College of Medicine; Faculty, Center for Female Pelvic Medicine and Reconstructive Surgery, Methodist Hospital/Clarian Health Partners; Urogynecology Associates, Indianapolis, Indiana

CONTENTS

Foreword   xiii
William F. Rayburn

Preface   xv
Rebecca G. Rogers

Surgical Education for the Twenty-First Century:
Beyond the Apprentice Model   233
Andrew J. Walter

> Traditionally, surgery has been taught by an apprentice model, where
> the learner imitates the actions of a skilled mentor. Although effective,
> this model is inefficient because it requires learners to be exposed to
> a large number of surgeries performed by a limited number of dedi-
> cated teaching faculty. In addition, competence is proved with sub-
> jective evaluations. Because of changes in modern medical practice,
> specifically reimbursement issues, resident work hour restrictions,
> and need for reliable and valid credentials, the critical components of
> the apprentice model are eroding. A paradigm shift is needed in mod-
> ern surgical education.

Changing the Way We Train Gynecologic Surgeons   237
Thomas M. Julian and Robert M. Rogers, Jr

> To ensure the integrity of gynecologic surgical practices and patient
> safety, changes need to be made in the training of gynecologic
> surgeons, both in residency and continuing surgical education.
> Although society demands competency in the training and contin-
> uing education of airline pilots, little is done in comparison to
> ensure competency in the training and continuing education of

gynecologic surgeons. Both professions rely on safe performance to protect the well-being of individuals. It is now time for medical and surgical education to move from the shadows of its "trust me" attitude into the light of a "test me and prove me" criterion.

Implementing a Surgical Skills Training Program   247
Robert A. Starr and Nathan V. Wagstaff

Significant change is underway in surgical training programs. Many educators believe that an outcomes-based approach to surgical education best addresses the need for greater public accountability and patient safety in surgical education. To achieve this end, surgical educators need to understand the basic principles of curriculum design and demonstrate a willingness to apply these educational methods within their training programs.

The Objective Structured Assessment of Technical Skills and the ACGME Competencies   259
Carmen J. Sultana

Objective structured assessment of technical skills is structured operating room or laboratory assessment of residents' surgical skills. It can be used to evaluate and teach both basic and complex skills to residents. The literature on its use is reviewed. Future use of virtual reality simulators is discussed.

From the Simple to the Sublime: Incorporating Surgical Models into Your Surgical Curriculum   267
Patrick J. Woodman and Charles W. Nager

Financial and time constraints have limited graduating residents' operative experience, making the use of models a necessary adjunct to a complete surgical curriculum. Models are useful tools to teaching surgical skills outside the operating room. They can be very realistic and complex, or they can be simple and economical. Models are developed to represent the anatomic arrangements seen in human patients, and to reproduce the biomechanical tasks necessary to complete a surgical case. Bench model laboratories are well-received by trainees and steepen the learning curve in the operating room.

Simulators and Virtual Reality in Surgical Education   283
Betty Chou and Victoria L. Handa

This article explores the pros and cons of virtual reality simulators, their abilities to train and assess surgical skills, and their potential future applications. Computer-based virtual reality simulators and more conventional box trainers are compared and contrasted. The virtual reality simulator provides objective assessment of surgical skills and immediate feedback further to enhance training. With this ability to provide standardized, unbiased assessment of surgical skills, the virtual reality trainer has the potential to be a tool for selecting, instructing, certifying, and recertifying gynecologists.

Mental Practice and Acquisition of Motor Skills: Examples from Sports Training and Surgical Education
Rebecca G. Rogers

297

Learning surgical skills involves both fine and gross motor skills, and necessitates performance in stressful situations. This environment is similar to the environment in which an athlete performs. Mental imagery has been used successfully in training athletes of all levels of proficiency and enhances both motor skills and motivational skills of performing under stress. The literature of using mental imagery to train surgeons is limited to the teaching of simple surgical skills, but shows promise as another tool to teach technical skills.

Teaching and Evaluating Ultrasound Skill Attainment: Competency-Based Resident Ultrasound Training for AIUM Accreditation
Rebecca Hall, Tony Ogburn, and Rebecca G. Rogers

305

Modern obstetrics and gynecology practice requires the frequent use of ultrasound and ultrasound training as a required component of obstetrics and gynecology residencies. Although programs do offer training in obstetric ultrasound imaging, education in gynecologic imaging is either absent or limited. This article describes a comprehensive ultrasound curriculum for obstetrics and gynecology residents that has been developed and implemented at the University of New Mexico. The curriculum is competency based and qualifies the graduating resident to seek American Institute of Ultrasound in Medicine laboratory accreditation.

How to Teach and Evaluate Learners in the Operating Room
Kimberly Kenton

325

The operating room is the universally established forum for learning surgical skills. It is the least structured and studied format, however, for teaching surgery. Establishing mutual, clear goals and expectations with residents or fellows before each case and reviewing their performance immediately after the case maximizes learning in the operating room.

Avoiding Pitfalls: Lessons in Surgical Teaching   **333**
Dee E. Fenner

> Becoming a good surgical educator takes time, patience, and dedication. Providing effective feedback is essential to improving the mentee's surgical skills. The operating room is a costly, high-risk classroom. Residents must come to the operating room prepared. Using a surgical skills laboratory can help in that preparation but is only effective when feedback is given regarding performance. While in the operating room, the attending physician must constantly direct, critique, and actively teach.

Index   **343**

FORTHCOMING ISSUES

September 2006
Thrombophilia and Women's Health
Isaac Blickstein, MD, *Guest Editor*

December 2006
Sexual Dysfunction
J. Chris Carey, MD, *Guest Editor*

RECENT ISSUES

March 2006
Myomas
Aydin Arici, MD, *Guest Editor*

December 2005
Cancer Complicating Pregnancy
Kimberly K. Leslie, MD, *Guest Editor*

September 2005
Preterm Labor: Prediction and Treatment
John C. Morrison, MD, *Guest Editor*

The Clinics are now available online!
http://www.theclinics.com

Obstet Gynecol Clin N Am
33 (2006) xiii–xiv

OBSTETRICS AND
GYNECOLOGY
CLINICS
OF NORTH AMERICA

Foreword

Teaching and Evaluating Surgical Skills

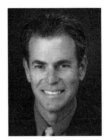

William F. Rayburn, MD
Consulting Editor

Gynecologic surgery has advanced during the past two decades. Refinements in instrumentation, video technology, suture material, and adhesion prevention have resulted in less morbid and more efficient procedures. New vistas will certainly challenge the new resident physician or the experienced surgeon to rethink his or her surgical approach. Cutting-edge robotics may forecast a time when the pelvic surgeon operates with accuracy and safety "away" from the patient. With the introduction of these new procedures and with more emphasis on quality assurance, there is a need to critically evaluate the surgeon's capabilities.

Dr. Rebecca Rogers guest edits a compelling issue dedicated to teaching and evaluating current skills while recognizing certain pitfalls to avoid in surgical training. This effort was undertaken in response to rapid changes encountered in the teaching of surgical principles. New surgical trainees and established surgeons alike will benefit from learning new technical approaches to prepare for evolving technology.

This issue reflects not only the basic, sound principles of established gynecologic surgical skills, but also what is controversial in the sometimes slow yet steady advance in knowledge of our surgical specialty. Major educational topics are addressed by the 15 contributing authors who excel as surgical educators. Uses of imagery and virtual reality simulations are presented along with specific suggestions for improving current techniques in the operating room. This com-

doi:10.1016/j.ogc.2006.02.006
obgyn.theclinics.com

pilation will serve students of all levels of experience with a structured assessment of their surgical skills.

William F. Rayburn, MD
Department of Obstetrics and Gynecology
University of New Mexico
MSC 10 5580
1 University of New Mexico
Albuquerque, NM 87131-0001, USA
E-mail address: wrayburn@salud.unm.edu

ELSEVIER
SAUNDERS

Obstet Gynecol Clin N Am
33 (2006) xv–xvi

OBSTETRICS AND
GYNECOLOGY
CLINICS
OF NORTH AMERICA

Preface

Teaching and Evaluating Surgical Skills

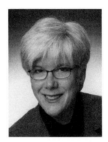

Rebecca G. Rogers, MD
Guest Editor

Surgical education is changing. Mandates that foster this change include increasing demands from the public for perfection without practice, decreasing trainee work hours, increasing minimally invasive therapies, and fewer surgical educators. In addition, rising health care costs have caused many experienced surgeons to focus on patient care rather than the mentoring of surgical trainees. A paradigm shift in surgical education is being forced by all these issues. This paradigm shift is important not only for new surgical trainees but also for established surgeons who need to learn new technical skills to keep pace with evolving medical technology and new procedures.

How can one ensure that the first time a trainee picks up a knife and makes an incision that he or she is as prepared to do so as possible? The apprenticeship model of surgical education, although time honored, falls short in proving competency and requires vast repetition to work. Animate and inanimate models, virtual reality, mental imagery, and the gold standard of attending teaching in the operating room will all likely play a role in surgical education of the future. Practice makes perfect and surgery, like any other technical skill, has to be practiced to become effortless. Few would argue that flight simulators are a sufficient proxy for flying an aircraft, but they are certainly better than no practice whatsoever. Technical skills, however, do not improve with practice without knowledgeable feedback, underlining the need for technical skills curricula that give trainees the opportunity to practice in a safe environment with adequate feedback.

0889-8545/06/$ – see front matter © 2006 Elsevier Inc. All rights reserved.
doi:10.1016/j.ogc.2006.02.002

obgyn.theclinics.com

Adequate measures to determine trainee competency are needed to ensure that when trainees are on their own, both their patients and employers know that they have not only completed their training but are also competent.

The inspiration for this edition of *Obstetrics and Gynecology Clinics of North America* arose out of a desire by the Education Committee of the American Urogynecology Society to improve surgical education in gynecology. Limitations of the Halstedian model of surgical education are reviewed, as are the ethics of surgical education. Presented is the limited literature that exists regarding the use of models, imagery, and virtual reality, and suggestions for improving surgical teaching in the operating room. The use of validated measures to evaluate surgical competency are also presented. The desire was to build on the excellent education we received as trainees and discuss limitations of what we experienced, with an eye to the future of surgical education in a changing landscape. It is hoped that this edition proves useful to surgical educators as they teach.

Rebecca G. Rogers, MD

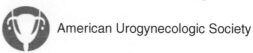 American Urogynecologic Society

Department of Obstetrics and Gynecology
University of New Mexico Health Sciences Center
Albuquerque, NM 87131, USA
E-mail address: rrogers@salud.unm.edu

ELSEVIER
SAUNDERS

Obstet Gynecol Clin N Am
33 (2006) 233–236

OBSTETRICS AND
GYNECOLOGY
CLINICS
OF NORTH AMERICA

Surgical Education for the Twenty-first Century: Beyond the Apprentice Model

Andrew J. Walter, MD

Division of Urogynecology, TPMG–Sacramento, 1650 Response Road, Sacramento, CA 95815, USA

Since the eighteenth century, as surgery evolved from a trade into a profession, the surgical education paradigm has been the apprentice model. This time-honored approach has remained the standard of practice to the present day. In this model, surgery is taught by the student directly observing and then imitating the actions of a skilled mentor [1]. Several critical factors are required to produce skilled surgeons in this model [2]: (1) a high volume of cases with multiple opportunities for repetition, (2) skilled surgical mentors and teachers, and (3) long work hours.

The apprentice model remains the current standard for surgical teaching. More importantly, most surgical teachers were the product of an apprenticeship system. This model produces competent if not somewhat jaded surgeons, both from overwork and the perceived or real abuse at the hands of mentors [2].

Goals of surgical education

Regardless of which model of education is used, the goals of surgical education should remain constant: to create competent surgeons [3]. Arguably, the component parts of a competent surgeon include all of the following [4]:

1. Knowledge: High order baseline knowledge regarding surgical anatomy, physiology, and disease processes
2. Leadership: Excellent leadership skills to maintain the proper flow and cohesiveness of the surgical team
3. Decision making: The ability to make critical decisions accurately and quickly

---

E-mail address: andrew.j.walter@kp.org

doi:10.1016/j.ogc.2006.01.003

4. Technical skills and dexterity (generally considered to be the most important factor): This is so that the surgical procedure can be completed with "elegance, efficiency and economy of movement" (J.F. Magrina, MD, personal communication, 1997). Skills and dexterity can be difficult to teach because gaining technical skill requires many innate characteristics, such as visuospatial recognition (the ability to see and process information in three dimensions) [5]; somatosensory memory (the key component to "see one, do one, teach one" [eg, the ability easily to remember and apply manual steps]); and stress tolerance.

The training of surgeons requires not only new effective methods of teaching surgical skills but also methods to assess whether the "taught" skills predict real world outcomes. Evaluative tools are needed that are both valid and reliable. This is paramount, because it is critical for both the newly graduated surgeon's patients and colleagues to be comfortable that the physician presented to them on paper is in fact a competent surgeon. Before discussing how this is done in the apprentice model, one first needs to understand the concepts of validity and reliability.

Validity and reliability

There are four major types of validity important to the interpretation of surgical evaluations.

1. Construct: Extent to which a test measures what it is supposed to measure or if a test discriminates between expertise levels. An example is, for the CREGO examinations to have construct validity, generally a chief resident should perform better than a junior resident on the test.
2. Predictive: The ability of an examination to predict future performance. An example is, does a high score on the CREOG examinations predict surgical excellence?
3. Face: The extent to which an examination mimics real situations. An example is, peeling the skin off of a grape in a laparoscopic model predicts how a resident will perform during a laparoscopic ovarian cystectomy.
4. Content: The extent to which the domain that is being measured is measured by the examination. An example is, do knowledge-based examinations, such as the Medical College Admission Test or National Board tests, measure technical dexterity?

Reliability is the extent to which a test generates similar results at two or more measurement points. There are three major facets of reliability to be considered during surgical assessment:

1. Test-retest: Do examinations given back-to-back give the same or similar results each time?

2. Interobserver: Do different observers give similar evaluations to the same resident?
3. Intraobserver: Does the same observer at different times give similar results to the same resident (assuming no intervention was done to improve the residents' performance)?

The good, the bad, and the ugly of the apprentice model

In the apprentice model, surgery is primarily taught by example with "see one, do one, then teach one" as the primary mode of knowledge acquisition. The apprentice model is clearly time honored, and it has been the model used for the entire history modern surgical practice. It is proved to work, in that most surgeons practicing today are all products of this system and are performing surgically in a successful fashion. In addition, by mentoring and behavioral modeling, the resident can learn the art of practicing medicine, something difficult to learn from textbooks or measure on examinations [6]. Unfortunately, as the complexity of surgical care and the constraints on teaching increase, it is increasingly difficult for teachers to function in the apprentice model. There are three specific areas of concern: (1) assessment of competency, (2) inefficiencies and time limitations inherent with mentor-dependent teaching, and (3) methods of credentialing.

Primarily competency is assessed by mentor-dependent ratings and written examinations (CREOGS, Boards). Secondary ratings may include surgical logbooks to document operative experience and morbidity and mortality reports to uncover complication rates or areas of potential patient mismanagement. Subjective mentor- dependent ratings of competency have numerous deficiencies with poor intraobserver and test-retest reliability and construct and predictive validity. Whether a good score on an evaluation is based on the skill of the ratee or how much the rater likes the ratee is difficult to determine. Written examinations, log books, and morbidity and mortality reports are more objective, assuming consistent inclusion criteria, and more reliable but suffer from poor validity. For example, written examinations assume that high test scores equals high technical proficiency and log books assume repetitive performance equals proficiency. Both of these evaluative methods have poor content and face validity. In addition, morbidity and mortality reports may reflect patient characteristics rather than poor performance, and have poor content validity.

Inefficiencies in the apprenticeship model of surgical training include gradually decreasing but generally intensive supervision, long resident hours to ensure adequate case exposure, and an approximate 1:1 ratio of residents and faculty. In modern medical practice, these factors are becoming increasingly difficult to provide because of two main issues. The first is resident work hour restrictions limited to 55 hours per week in Europe and 80 hours per week in the United States [7,8]. This represents a 20% to 50% decrease in residency length based on hours spent in the hospital and reduces the exposure of residents to their surgical mentors. The second is the realities of the business of medicine. Because of changes in reimbursement and other insurance and medicolegal issues, there is less opportunity for "teachers to teach" [9]. Specific issues include productivity constraints, need for timely completion of the surgical procedure, and patient safety concerns.

In the current system, there are two main requirements to attain postresidency credentialing to practice surgery. The first is completion of an accredited residency program. The second is to pass a series of written and oral examinations. These tend to have poor validity or reliability for the prediction of surgical competence and likely become even more so as residency hours are further reduced and staff productivity constraints become more problematic.

A good model requiring change: conclusion

To keep the apprentice model as the primary method for the surgical education of residents, three things need to be modified from the current situation: (1) changing Medicare reimbursement procedures to account for teaching time, (2) improving salaries for academic faculty to encourage greater participation in academic medicine and improve the resident and faculty ratios, and (3) making residency training longer. Quite frankly, none of these are likely to occur.

A new paradigm for surgical education is now needed, and this requires a new model for education. It is important to realize, however, that the apprenticeship model will never entirely be removed from surgical education and that mentors are required to teach the art of surgery. What is needed, in addition to skilled mentors, are more efficient methods of teaching and more objective methods of assessment. The goal of these new methods, discussed elsewhere in this issue, is consistently to produce qualified surgeons with reliable and valid credentials.

References

[1] Dunnington GL. The art of mentoring. Am J Surg 1996;171:604–7.
[2] Wolfe JH. General surgical training: improvements and problems. Ann R Coll Surg Engl 1998; 80(3 Suppl):112–6.
[3] Sachdeva AK. Acquisition and maintenance of surgical competence. Semin Vasc Surg 2002;15: 182–90.
[4] Hamdorf JM, Hall JC. Acquiring surgical skills. Br J Surg 2000;87:28–37.
[5] Rissuci DA. Visual spatial perception and surgical competence. Am J Surg 2002;184:291–5.
[6] Marckmann G. Teaching science vs. the apprentice model: do we really have the choice? Med Health Care Philos 2001;4:85–9.
[7] Kort KC, Pavone LE, Jenson E, et al. Resident perceptions of the impact of work hour restrictions on health care delivery and surgical education: time for a transformational change. Surgery 2004;136:861–71.
[8] Winslow ER, Bowman MC, Klingensmith ME, et al. Surgeon workhours in the era of limited workhours. J Am Coll Surg 2004;198:111–7.
[9] Sakorafas GH, Tsiotos GC. New legislative regulations, problems and future perspectives, with a particular emphasis on surgical education. J Postgrad Med 2004;50:274–7.

ELSEVIER
SAUNDERS

Obstet Gynecol Clin N Am
33 (2006) 237–246

OBSTETRICS AND
GYNECOLOGY
CLINICS
OF NORTH AMERICA

Changing the Way We Train Gynecologic Surgeons

Thomas M. Julian, MD[a,*], Robert M. Rogers, Jr, MD[b]

[a]Department of Obstetrics and Gynecology, University of Wisconsin Medical School,
Clinical Science Center, H4/646, 600 Highland Avenue, Madison, WI 53792, USA
[b]Northwest Women's Health Center, 75 Claremont Street A, Kalispell, Montana 59901-3500, USA

Less than 75 years ago in the United States, the training of the gynecologic surgeon relied on apprenticeship. This model was variable in training time, surgical cases performed, and skills acquired. The system was a "see one, do one, teach one" from mentor to student, passed down through professional generations. In his 1910 report on medical education in the United States and Canada, Flexner [1] wrote, "We have indeed in America medical practitioners not inferior to the best elsewhere; but there is probably no other country in the world in which there is so great a distance and so fatal a difference between the best, the average, and the worst." Flexner continued, "The examination for licensure is indubitably the lever with which the entire field may be lifted; for the power to examine is the power to destroy...bad teaching, lack of clinical material, failure to correlate laboratory and clinic...." He concluded that a poorly trained candidate "would be detected and punished by a searching practical examination."

In 1924, Lynch [2] suggested gynecologic surgery trainees should be exposed to 1500 to 2000 surgical cases and "actually perform all the work in 150 or more major gynecologic cases, which are selected to present all types of our more serious problems....Not the least important feature of the plan is the opportunity afforded the candidate to serve a long term in the follow-up clinic, through which he will learn the actual results obtained from treatment." The American Board of Obstetrics and Gynecology, founded in 1930, administered the first written, oral,

* Corresponding author.
E-mail address: tmjulian@wisc.edu (T.M. Julian).

0889-8545/06/$ – see front matter © 2006 Elsevier Inc. All rights reserved.
doi:10.1016/j.ogc.2006.01.005

clinical, and pathologic examinations to 79 applicants in 1931, certifying 65. These examinations were based on testing and review of clinical cases, as suggested [3].

Presently, American society and various government agencies are concerned about the continued reports of medical mistakes and the ever increasing cost of obtaining medical and surgical care. In response to these concerns, the Accreditation Council for Graduate Medical Education (ACGME), the governing body for postgraduate education, recommends changing graduate medical education from the "structure-and-process" model to an "educational outcomes" model to determine the clinical competency of each resident [4]. The structure-and-process model trains residents based on the number and types of lectures offered, and the clinical volume and experience available. These criteria are defined loosely and monitored by the Residency Review Committee (RRC) for Obstetrics and Gynecology, the enforcement arm of the ACGME. The clinical and surgical competency of each resident in the existing model, however, is in practice subjectively determined by the individual residency program director.

The ACGME proposed educational outcomes model, endorsed in 1997, suggests the competency of each resident be measured by rigorous, objective educational testing of clinical knowledge and surgical skills. The ACGME, the American Board of Medical Specialties, and the Accreditation Council on Continuing Medical Education have mandated that residents be trained to be competent in the following six areas: (1) patient care, (2) medical knowledge, (3) practice-based learning and improvement, (4) interpersonal and communication skills, (5) professionalism, and (6) systems-based practice. The competency-based teaching and testing of residents progressing through training are to be developed and based on reproducible, evidence-based models. Just as clinical decisions should be determined by evidence-based clinical studies in the literature, surgical training models, including testing, should be determined by evidence-based educational studies. Individuals are motivated to learn more when they know their knowledge and skills will be tested. Competency-based teaching and testing models need to be developed and standardized nationwide to establish uniformity in gynecologic surgical training. Competency-demonstrated curricula are a response to public demands to improve quality control in the teaching of medical and surgical services and to link accountability to the public funding of graduate medical education [5]. In addition, as American society and the legal system have evolved in the past 50 years, there is also a mandate, even less well defined, to evaluate the ethics involved in the training of medical clinicians and surgeons.

The current environment of training gynecologic surgeons

These proposed changes come at a time of a growing concern among experienced gynecologic surgeons in the United States that the newest members of the specialty are not being adequately trained nor evaluated for competency in clinical practice [6–10]. It is speculated that this concern results from several changes within and outside of the specialty and training programs. These factors are the decreasing volume and variety of teaching cases available to residents; the increasing numbers of new, minimally invasive procedures; the decreasing numbers of dedicated surgical instructors; and the instructor-based model of teaching surgery [10].

The decreasing number and variety of gynecologic procedures available for teaching are believed to be the result of four factors. First, many surgical diseases are now managed with medication, physical therapy, or counseling. Examples include chronic pelvic pain, urinary incontinence, endometriosis, infertility, abnormal uterine bleeding, fibroids, and ectopic pregnancy. Second, more limited-practice gynecologic surgeons, including endoscopists, infertility specialists, and reparative vaginal surgeons, are performing surgeries in competition with the same population of patients as the local residency programs. Third, increased curricular requirements and limitations of resident work hours leave less time for experience in surgery. Fourth, government and third-party payers decrease health care costs by arbitrarily requiring nonsurgical therapies in many cases by making surgical precertification difficult to obtain.

Increasing laparoscopic, hysteroscopic, and minimally invasive procedures add additional sets of skills with different instrumentation than traditional gynecologic surgery. These procedures require development of expert hand-eye coordination and fine motor skills along with the challenge of operating in the confines of a two-dimensional monitor view of the three-dimensional surgical field of the female pelvis.

The financial support available for teaching in departments of obstetrics and gynecology has significantly decreased in the past 15 years. As a result, the academic faculty is expected to spend more time in direct patient care to generate departmental revenue. Consequently, the faculty has less time for direct resident education. Many faculty members have chosen to retire early or to leave academics for more financially rewarding private practices. This also decreases the available surgical mentoring of younger teaching faculty. Many teachers in the specialty believe that there has been a significant decrease in the interaction of gynecology residents with experienced gynecologic surgeons.

Lastly, the present instructor-oriented style of teaching is still very subjective and may perpetuate poor surgical skills and decision-making at the operating table [6]. The resident is not learning skills and management based on evidence-based educational tools, but is learning based on the subjective experience of the mentor. When this is the case, surgical instruction has been shown to be random without goals and without valid measurement. The teaching is based on the instructor's own whims at that particular case. Surgical instruction at the table often is a "trial by exhaustion and humiliation, as well as a journey of harassment and abuse" [11]. Current residency guidelines contain no uniform standards for determining competency in surgical training, making surgical assessment subjective or nonexistent [12].

Ethics and surgical training

How do surgical instructors in gynecologic procedures approach the important task of training competent gynecologic surgeons for the future benefit of women's health care, while safeguarding the safety and personal dignity of each patient [13]? The answer must include guidelines for hands-on residency training and the development of a system of ethics for providing quality surgical care. This must also include the ethics of training experienced surgeons in performing new, innovative procedures not learned in residency. Residency training addresses "performing an accepted operation for the first time." Practitioner training addresses "performing a new operation for the first time." That is, devices and technologies should not be used until practitioners are sufficiently trained in their use to ensure quality patient care.

The ACGME has assigned "professionalism" as an area of core competency. This is defined as "a commitment to carrying out professional responsibilities, adherence to ethical principles, and sensitivity to patients of diverse backgrounds." Ethics, broadly defined, are the morality, beliefs, and values practiced by an individual. Ethics change as an individual and a society change. In the present-day practice of medicine and surgery in the United States, ethical considerations recommend management and procedures that produce the best result for each patient, while considering the needs of American society as a whole. Currently, "what is best" and "the needs of our society" include a mandate to decrease health care costs.

With all these factors considered, the goal of the surgical educator is to prepare each resident for the independent practice of surgery. This should occur after extensive preoperative skills training outside of the operating room, followed by progressive surgical experience under the direct supervision of a seasoned mentor. The patient should be informed that the surgery will be performed by both the teaching surgeon and the resident surgeon as a team [13]. Unfortunately, many residency programs do not plan for adequate surgical skills training before entering the operating room. Many residents begin learning their surgical skills at the time of actual surgery. In his article "Ethical Problems Special to Surgery," Moore [13] states, "The American residency system of postgraduate education fosters and institutionalizes these relationships to ensure the welfare of patients in a teaching environment." Is this always true? Is the surgeon-in-training prepared in a systematic, progressive manner?

The second ethical problem concerns gynecologic surgeons desiring to perform new surgical procedures. The surgeon must temper the excitement of "trying something new" with the moderating principles of "do no harm" and "what is truly best for the patient"? Preparatory work should be performed before introducing a new surgical procedure or device. Many innovative laparoscopic procedures, reparative vaginal procedures, and surgeries for stress urinary incontinence have been introduced and performed over the past 10 years. But have these procedures always been based on good evidence? Has effective training been planned, provided, and properly completed by each practitioner to ensure sufficient operator experience for patient safety and procedural efficacy?

Some new surgical techniques are driven by aggressive marketing by medical device manufacturers, including courses for surgeons, direct advertisements to patients, and media coverage. These newer procedures and devices are commonly advocated by well-known surgeons who see themselves as pioneers, but who also reap financial gain from their industry relationships. Even the present regulation of these new surgical techniques on the national level is suspect.

There are few randomized controlled trials of new surgical techniques or devices comparing them with the gold standard before they are introduced into practice. Most new devices are introduced on the basis of Food and Drug Administration (FDA) approval under the 510(k) exemption. The new device is approved under the claim that it is substantially equivalent to existing devices and should be exempt from further trials or FDA hearings. Most are approved. All 510(k) exemptions are public record [14] (http://www.accessdata.fda.gov/scripts/cdrh/cfdocs/cfPMN/pmn.cfm).

Many surgeons are motivated to learn new procedures based on the attitude of "Look what I can do" and "How can I better market myself"? The types of factors that drive a practitioner to be the first to introduce a new procedure to a community, especially without strong evidence of its worth, are seldom mentioned in surgical training courses. These motivations are suspect because using new surgical procedures, devices, or techniques in this manner does not put the patient first. Ideally, surgeons should think of their patients and consider safety, efficacy, cost, and his or her qualifications to perform the new technique. How does one teach and enforce this in practice?

The introduction of these new devices by manufacturers accounts for most surgical teaching for practicing gynecologists. The most common method of introducing and teaching these new surgical techniques is the industry-sponsored weekend crash course that financially benefits the manufacturer or distributor. Teaching methods at these seminars are variable and consist of handouts and lectures, which discuss indications, techniques, contraindications, complications, and problem management. Included is ample discussion for product placement. These techniques may be supplemented with videos, practice on inanimate models, live demonstrations on laboratory animals or human cadavers, or direct observations in the operating room [15].

These crash courses are unlike resident training, which is based on the principles of hands-on apprenticeship with increasing levels of complexity and appropriate mentoring and supervision. Training for the surgeon once in practice is not standardized, and in most cases, neither mentored nor monitored. Most hospitals and surgery centers have no formal method to ensure competency of a surgeon using a new technique. Experienced gynecologic surgeons should demonstrate four basic qualities before implementing new technology: (1) understanding of the anatomy and pathophysiology of the diseased organ or disease process, (2) knowledge of alternative medical or surgical therapies,

(3) ability to explain risks and benefits of a procedure to patients, and (4) awareness of self-limitations as a practitioner and as a surgeon.

As is stated by the ethics committee of the American College of Obstetricians and Gynecologists [16]:

> If health care professionals are to benefit society, they must be well educated and experienced. Acquisition of knowledge and skills in the educational process entails both benefits and risks. The benefits of health care to society provide the justification for exposure of patients to risks associated with education in clinical medicine. While the benefits generally accrue to society at large, the burdens fall primarily on individual patients, especially the economically disadvantaged. These burdens are inherent in situations in which patients interact with students, for example, during medical histories, physical examinations, and diagnostic and surgical procedures.
>
> Physicians must learn new skills and techniques in a manner consistent with the ethical obligations to benefit the patient, to do no harm, and to respect a patient's right to make informed decisions about health matters. These obligations must not be unjustifiably subordinated to the need and desire to learn new skills. In consideration of society's interest in the education of physicians, all patients should be considered 'teaching patents.' Race or socioeconomic status should not be the basis for selection of patients for teaching.

Postgraduate training, both in residency and postresidency, is monitored in poorly defined ways. The monitoring process is not well coordinated. Monitoring is performed by multiple committees, agencies, or organizations, including licensing authorities, voluntary national and state societies, and for most practitioners, most directly by local departmental and hospital practice committees. There is no assurance that teaching, learning, and practice in either setting meet any ethical standards. Presently, actions against physicians at any level of practice are based primarily on patient care outcomes. Usually litigation spurs this action. If a residency program or practitioner is following "standard of care" and "within the norm" at the occurrence of adverse patient outcomes, then compliance with ethical standards is assumed. Much harder to detect are surgeons performing unnecessary procedures without complications because the lack of complications fails to initiate a departmental review.

Two additional concerns in the ethical training of gynecologic surgeons need to be addressed. The first concerns how ethics are taught to residents. The second concerns the ethics of changing curricula of residency and postresidency education. The ACGME lists "professionalism" as one of its six areas of core competency. Professionalism is defined as "...a commitment to carrying out professional responsibilities, adherence to ethical principles, and sensitivity to patients diverse backgrounds." There are no further guidelines or clarifications. The determination of satisfactory completion of residency requirements and final competency for each obstetrics and gynecology resident trainee rests with the individual program director. The residency program director certifies that each graduating resident is sufficiently prepared and competent to pursue certification by the American Board of Obstetrics and Gynecology.

The Council on Resident Education in Obstetrics and Gynecology requirements beginning July, 2005, only reiterate the statement on professionalism, mentioning "ethics and medical jurisprudence" together under the section on "primary and preventive care." No further direction or clarification is given. For "gynecology" under the heading of "specific educational experiences," Council on Resident Education in Obstetrics and Gynecology educational objectives state only that the resident be competent in "the full range of medical and surgical gynecology for all age groups, including experience in the management of critically ill patients."

Concerning the ethics of the teachers in obstetrics and gynecology training, it is no secret that the residency program director fills out the RRC forms in the best possible light, having vested interest in program preservation, minimizing program revision, and graduating residents who have attended their program. In contrast, the RRC for many years has told the program directors that reviews can be used to help programs recognize and correct deficiencies. A RRC review can be used to improve and strengthen the quality of resident education and training. In actuality, program directors often coach the residents to avoid making negative comments to the RRC reviewers. Residency directors have been known to make residents believe that such negative comments may lead to an action that could jeopardize the continuation of the program and force the residents to transfer elsewhere to finish their training. Presently, residency completion is more a certificate of time served than a measure of education and skill attainment.

A proposal for training the gynecologic surgeon

Many gynecologic surgical educators believe that the surgical training of residents has suffered in the past 15 years and is insufficient for recent gynecology resident graduates to meet present-day practice standards [6–10]. The authors have proposed that gynecologic surgical education should be guided by evidence-based educational studies, just as clinical care should be guided by evidence-based clinical reports [10]. Surgical teaching outcomes should be measured in a reproducible manner. Surgical curriculum should be written to standardize core knowledge, surgical skills preparation, judgment involved in preoperative evaluation, intraoperative performance, treatment of complications, and postoperative management. The intangible qualities of ethics, professionalism, communication, and leadership should be integrated into training in a measurable way. These qualities require further study and definition to develop curricula, teaching techniques, and methods of evaluation. Patterns and habits of study and literature review must be taught to ensure the individual's future self-education as a board-certified, practicing surgical gynecologist. Above all, the education of enthusiastic, dedicated mentors is crucial to the progress toward competency-based excellence in training the gynecologic surgeon.

During training, the resident should perform a minimum number of required surgical procedures, with the surgical mentor documenting resident involvement in each case including decision making, and measurable, objective feedback on resident performance and progress. The course of instruction should include various learning activities to teach and practice basic surgical knowledge, patterns of decision making and leadership, and manual skills before the resident actually assists at his or her first case. This course may include readings, lectures, videos, discussions, observations of live surgeries, and practice on inanimate and animal practice models. The resident-in-training must be accountable for his or her own progress through the surgical curriculum. Mentor feedback needs to be immediate, frequent, and objective, yet supportive and encouraging. The mentor's evaluation should be verbal at the end of each case, and dictated or written for documentation and review of the resident's progress. This is as important as dictating the operative report or writing a progress note and allows for objective review over time by the resident and mentor, and the program director.

The acquisition of core surgical knowledge, judgment, leadership qualities, and skills before the resident participates in live surgeries is the keystone in fulfilling the mandate to improve the ethics and effectiveness of training gynecologic surgeons. The live surgeries on actual patients that the resident begins to participate in as an assistant should be those that are the most common and plentiful [17]. The gynecologic resident should proceed incrementally to surgical experiences with ever more increasing difficulty. Eventually, the resident operates as the primary surgeon with the mentor as the assistant.

Educators in the specialty who proscribe and oversee residency training should take this opportunity to reorganize and study objectively how best to train the future generations of gynecologic surgeons. Doing the best possible job in training is the most ethical practice model that can be provided. This example in itself results in self-motivation and self-direction for future learning by the graduated gynecologic surgeon.

Time in training should be increased to 5 years [10]. The authors propose that the PGY-1 or first year in an obstetrics and gynecology residency be a well-defined and supervised transitional year of primary care medicine and basic surgical learning. The PGY-2 to PGY-4 years should be a 36-month experience to learn the presentation and management of the most common problems in obstetrics, gynecology, and gynecologic surgery. This time should also involve rotations through the clinical subspecialties of obstetrics and gynecology to learn the thought processes and approaches to the management of the more complex patients. In the authors' opinion, the current program curriculum that divides training time equally among obstetric and gynecologic rotations needs to be rethought and revised. The present training time allotted for residents to perform hundreds of normal, spontaneous vaginal deliveries needs to be revisited. Time for resident training should be influenced by the requirements of the evolving subspecialty clinical areas, many of which did not exist when current training requirements were formulated.

The PGY-5 year should be a transition period from residency to independent practice or further postgraduate training. In this fifth year, the resident should be a minimally supervised junior faculty member and assist in teaching, evaluating, and supervising the PGY-2 to PGY-4 residents. The best way to master a subject is to practice and teach it. At the same time, the PGY-5 resident should generate case lists and experiences directly leading to board certification immediately at the satisfactory completion of residency.

The authors propose that a few residency programs in obstetrics and gynecology around the United States be designated and funded to study the best methods of teaching gynecologic surgery. These centers should develop curricula, teaching methods, testing tools, and standards of evaluation that are evidence-based. The primary goal of these centers is to give the RRC an objective, tested program to evaluate and certify all residency training. Ideally, public and private payers of health care, national foundations, and specialty societies should be included in this process. Funding support and intellectual input for these centers should be seen as a benefit to payers, medical educators, and patients by providing competency-based training and practices. The result to society and individual patients is competent gynecologic surgeons with a commitment to excellence in learning and in assimilating the true advances in the practice of obstetrics, gynecology, and surgery. These gynecologic practitioners will have demonstrated competency in knowledge, skills, judgment, leadership, integrity, and high ethical values.

For the teaching of new surgical techniques to gynecologists already in practice, the authors propose that FDA approval of a new procedure or device also include the submission of an effective model of teaching surgeons on how safely to perform the procedure or use the new device. This should include seminars with testing objectives, instructional models with demonstrations, and meaningful mentoring by qualified experts in the field. Input for the FDA on the new procedure and device, and in effective training, should be required from unbiased, recognized experts, and not from those surgeons with financial interests in the product or its profits. Without such approval from the FDA and without documentation of sufficient surgical training, no surgeon should be credentialed or allowed to perform the new procedure or use the new device.

Summary

If the integrity of gynecologic surgical practices and patient safety are going to be ensured, changes need to be made in the training of gynecologic surgeons, both in residency and continuing surgical education. Although society demands competency in training and continuing education of airline pilots, little is done in comparison to ensure competency in training and continuing education of gynecologic surgeons. Both professions rely on safe performance to protect the well-being of individuals. It is now time for medical and surgical education to move from the shadows of its "trust me" attitude into the light of a "test me and prove me" criterion.

References

[1] Flexner A. Medical education in the United States and Canada: a report to the Carnegie Foundation for the Advancement of Teaching. New York: The Carnegie Foundation for the Advancement of Teaching. Bull. No. 4, 1910.

[2] Lynch F. The specialty of gynecology and obstetrics. JAMA 1924;83:397–9.

[3] Speert H. Obstetrics and gynecology in America: a history. Chicago: The American College of Obstetricians and Gynecologists; 1980.

[4] American Urogynecologic Society. Using outcomes to evaluate surgical competency: a new model for graduate medical education. AUGS Quarterly Report 2003;22:1–4.

[5] Carraccio C, Wolfsthal SD, Englander R, et al. Shifting paradigms: from Flexner to competencies. Acad Med 2002;77:361–7.

[6] Mandel LP, Lentz GM, Goff BA. Teaching and evaluating surgical skills. Obstet Gynecol 2000;95:783–5.

[7] Sorosky JL, Anderson B. Surgical experiences and training of residents: perspectives of experienced gynecologic oncologists. Gynecol Oncol 1999;75:222–3.

[8] Julian TM. The training of gynecologic surgeons. J Pelvic Med Surg 2003;9:179–87.

[9] Rogers Jr RM. Training the gynecologic surgeon. In: Rock JA, Jones III HW, editors. TeLinde's operative gynecology. Philadelphia: Lippincott Williams & Wilkins; 2003. p. 1561–7.

[10] Rogers Jr RM, Julian TM. Training the gynecologic surgeon. Obstet Gynecol 2005;105: 197–200.

[11] Dunnington GL. The art of mentoring. Am J Surg 1996;171:604–7.

[12] General and special requirements for graduate medical education. Chicago: Accreditation Council for Graduate Medical Education; 2002.

[13] Moore FD. Ethical problems special to surgery. Arch Surg 2000;135:14–6.

[14] Tolomeo DE. The use of Food and Drug Administration 510(k) notifications in patient litigation. Food Drug Law J 2004;59:465–71.

[15] Udwadia TE. Guidelines for laparoscopic surgery. Indian Journal of Medical Ethics 1997;5(2). Available at: http://www.issueinmedicalethics.org/052mi040.html.

[16] American College of Obstetricians and Gynecologists. Ethical issues in obstetric-gynecologic education. In: Ethics in obstetrics and gynecology. Washington: ACOG; 2000. p. 35–7.

[17] Brill AI, Rogers Jr RM. A new paradigm for resident training [editorial]. J Am Assoc Gynecol Laparosc 1998;5:219–20.

ELSEVIER
SAUNDERS

Obstet Gynecol Clin N Am
33 (2006) 247–258

OBSTETRICS AND
GYNECOLOGY
CLINICS
OF NORTH AMERICA

Implementing a Surgical Skills Training Program

Robert A. Starr, MD*, Nathan V. Wagstaff, MD

*Department of Obstetrics and Gynecology, William Beaumont Hospital, 3601 West 13 Mile Road,
Royal Oak, MI 48073–6769, USA*

Surgery is responsibility

Francis D. Moore, MD, Harvard Medical School

Patients consent for surgery based upon trust, a trust that the surgeon is sufficiently experienced to exercise sound judgment and technically competent to execute the task at hand. Surgical competence is difficult to define. Several authors have recently addressed the challenging question of "What makes a surgeon competent?" and in so doing, have concluded that surgical competence is the product of multiple factors, including adequate core medical knowledge, good clinical decision-making skills and judgment, professionalism, keen interpersonal and communication skills, and technical expertise [1–3]. As academic surgeons, teaching surgical technical skills is one of the most important responsibilities.

A changing landscape

This past decade represents one of the most dynamic times in surgical education because surgical teachers have been challenged to question traditional educational approaches [4]. Two forces that have led to consensus for changing surgical education are the realization that the ultimate technical skills of a trainee cannot easily be predicted on matriculation into a training program and that the

---

* Corresponding author.
E-mail address: rstarr@beaumont.edu (R.A. Starr).

traditional Halstedian apprenticeship method may be too subjective and unreliable to predict future surgical competence. Additionally, regulatory duty hour restrictions, medical economic cost containment, competing curriculum content, and initiatives that address societal and medicolegal concerns, including efforts to reduce medical errors, all add to the drive to reshape surgical skills education. In the United States, change has been driven primarily by the Accreditation Council for Graduate Medical Education *Outcomes Project*, an approach to resident education that moves away from the traditional emphasis on training program structure and process and toward a competency-based approach. This newer philosophic focus is characterized by the underlying principles that whatever one measures, one tends to improve, and that patient and public accountability are better served by focusing on the ultimate measure of surgical competence, namely clinical outcomes [5].

Although not without significant challenges, an outcomes-focused approach to determining surgical competence has distinct advantages as outlined by Ritchie [6]. Specifically, clinical outcomes are likely the best measure of competence because they are definable, easily discovered and reviewed, and serve as a reasonable proxy to other elements of competence including technical skills, cognitive ability, and clinical decision-making. In addition, national norms for surgical outcomes can be or in some instances are already established.

Teaching technical skills is a core component of any surgery-based residency. Increasing numbers of residency programs are establishing outcomes-based education, and in so doing, linking their educational learning objectives to meaningful, valid, and reliable evidence that their curricular objectives are being achieved. When implementing a surgical skills teaching program, it is important to keep in mind that "education" and "training" are inseparable and both are necessary [7]. In the past, medical education has largely occurred through self-directed or assigned reading, lectures, and interactive teaching sessions. Interactive teaching sessions have been shown to be superior to didactic teaching in several areas of study [8]. Despite this observation, didactic teaching will likely continue to play a large role in medical education because of practical considerations, such as time availability and resource allocation. In contrast, technical skills training has taken place in the operating room, in the context of caring for live patients. Although this time-honored approach will continue to comprise a significant portion of surgical training, there is increasing interest in and reliance on lower-stakes and less resource-intensive supplemental educational experiences. Understanding these methods and incorporating them is one key to developing a surgical skills curriculum successfully.

Getting started

Some key concepts are essential to developing an effective surgical skills teaching program, including understanding how students learn technical skills. DesCoteaux and Leclere [9] provide an excellent review of how motor skills are learned. In their thoughtful overview paper, the authors detail the basic elements of several learning theories and their implications for surgical skills learning and instruction. Surgical students must possess the prerequisites of sufficient knowledge, sound judgment, and a professional attitude before starting a curriculum. Ideally, both learner and teacher should embrace certain adult learning principles. Instruction should be learner-centered, self-directed, and focused on applicable real world tasks that affect the learner's experience in a way that motivates him or her to pursue the educational experience. The authors further point out that basic surgical skills are linked in the operating room into an orderly series or interplay of steps commonly referred to as "executive routines." These routines are the product of learning the fundamental technical skills and linking them in more sophisticated patterns or hierarchies.

To develop and implement a surgical skills training program effectively, educators must also be familiar with other key elements of teaching technical 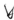 skills: (1) to identify the fundamental technical and ergonomic skills to be learned, (2) to provide the knowledge base for understanding the technical skills, (3) to define exercises to practice the skills, (4) to teach and model perfect execution of the skills, (5) to create opportunities for supervised practice, (6) to develop methods for evaluation and feedback, and (7) to develop a curriculum that ties the elements together. This article expands on these elements to provide a guide to the steps of how to implement a surgical skills teaching program.

The curriculum

A curriculum is defined as a particular course of study, often in a special field. The curriculum serves both as a map detailing the educational destination and a compass providing the direction or instructional plan for achieving the end point. In the case of surgical skills training, the end point is independent performance of surgery. A curriculum is more than just a series of topics and exercises or a syllabus; it is a plan that is comprehensive and cohesive, providing both instructional scope and sequence beginning with an educational end in mind.

A curriculum contains many parts, all of which relate to the end objective of developing a comprehensive plan to achieve a specific educational goal. The components of a well-designed curriculum include

1. Goals: the educational outcomes or desired real world performance; they define the curricular content
2. Terminal objectives: describe in precise, measurable terms what the learners will be able to do at the end of an instructional sequence
3. Instructional strategies: the ways in which the curricular objectives will be met
4. Evaluation strategies: methods to determine if the learners have achieved the terminal objectives

5. Curriculum management and implementation plan: divides the curriculum into tasks and defines the necessary resources and represents an overarching matrix encompassing all the prior steps

Needs assessment

An important first step in curriculum development is performing a needs assessment. This is a systematic process to determine what educational solutions close the gap between what target learners currently know and do and what they need to know and do. A needs assessment can be accomplished through any of a number of steps, including informal or structured query of current residents and teaching faculty or a survey of former graduates to assess where their education could have been strengthened. The process demands that the individual responsible for overseeing the teaching of surgical skills is thoroughly familiar with the program-specific requirements issued by the specialty accreditation body. In doing so, an inventory of what must be taught becomes the minimum basis for the ultimate curriculum.

Rationale statement

Any meaningful curriculum requires many resources ranging from faculty, physical space to conduct instructional exercises, learning supplies or materials, and both dedicated teaching and learning time in the overall training curriculum. Each of these carries with it a value, the cost of which must be supported to succeed in the teaching effort. To argue successfully for such support, it may be necessary to follow the needs assessment process with writing of a curricular development rationale statement. The rationale statement usually expresses the curriculum developer's beliefs and understanding about the importance of the learning material and explains the educational purpose of the curriculum. Key questions should be addressed in the statement, such as "What educational problems are targeted?," "What changes prompt the curriculum development?," "Why is the curriculum important to the learners?," and "Who are the anticipated beneficiaries of the curriculum?." By detailing this information, it becomes easier to garner administrative support and the rationale statement (Box 1) itself becomes a guiding document for the ongoing curricular process.

Curricular design

The various components of curricular design interrelate to support the desired end product, which can be termed the "educational goals or outcomes" (Fig. 1). In the case of surgical skills training, the principle educational outcome is the competent performance of surgery. It is this end point that drives the curriculum. By beginning with the desired goal in mind, the curriculum becomes the composite of steps necessary to achieve that goal. A brief review of these basic steps follows.

Box 1. Example rational statement

Many factors impact contemporary teaching of surgical skills including time constraints, fiscal pressures, societal and ethical considerations, increasing complexity of some surgical procedures, and stricter expectations by oversight organizations. As surgical education evolves, there is an increasing need to include supplemental learning opportunities outside the operating room. Therefore, the need exists to develop a surgical skills training laboratory with an accompanying formal curriculum. It is expected that trainees will enhance their learning of basic surgical skills and benefit through better preparation for the operating room experience.

Determining educational goals

Although curriculum design can be approached in multiple ways, many educators begin by asking "What do we want our learners to be able to do when they are done?," and then determine the terminal or learning objectives and corresponding teaching techniques to support these educational goals. This method of reverse design identifies the goals or desired results and next determines the level of acceptable evidence to support achievement of the goals. Viewed this way, the basic model can be applied to any level of curricular content. For instance, if the end goal is that the learner competently closes an abdominal incision, several subordinate goals comprise the learning experience. These may include recall of abdominal wall anatomy, appropriate suture selection, and the technical execution

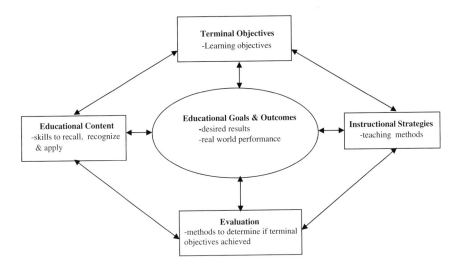

Fig. 1. Curricular design.

of knot tying and suturing. Each subordinate goal then has a corresponding evaluation method to confirm achievement of the desired outcome, and in turn an appropriately assigned instructional strategy or learning method.

Developing terminal (learning) objectives

Learning objectives become the essential means for delineating the educational goals or desired outcomes. Objectives clarify exactly what residents are expected to know and do, providing detail to both the learner and teacher. Learning objectives should be written in measurable behavioral terms. Because in the reverse design method of curriculum development the metrics and standards for learner performance are predetermined, the learning objectives guide the instructors toward meaningful evaluation techniques.

To develop learning objectives, curriculum developers must specify certain key details. For example, the objectives should state the level of expertise of the learner (eg, PGY-1 resident); what the learner will be able to do (behavior or action verb combined with curriculum content or goal); the condition or circumstance in which the learner is to perform; and the standard or benchmark the learner is expected to achieve. The combination of these essential elements provides the direction for instructional strategies and evaluation techniques.

Choosing instructional strategies

Instructional strategies are comprised of the ways in which the terminal or learning objectives are taught. Exactly what will be taught should already be framed by the target educational goals and learning objectives. Choosing the teaching methods should address the question of what activities best equip a given level of learner with the target knowledge or skills.

Because of expanding curricular content in residency education, competition for instructional time is a pressing reality in most training programs. This forces teachers to consider educational content and teaching time and methods in the context of levels of curricular priority. The less time allotted to a given teaching session, the greater the focus on the information that provides enduring understanding of a topic and the more honed an instructional strategy should be to achieve the specific educational goal. Aside from time, careful consideration must also be given to what faculty and material resources are necessary for a given instructional method.

In addition to giving priority to essential ideas, faculty should consider other key principles when designing a curriculum including (1) providing meaningfulness or a real world link of the content to surgical practice; (2) communicating all prerequisites for a teaching session, such as reading or practice assignments; (3) using learning aids and, when appropriate, novelty to teach; (4) modeling, especially when addressing technical skills; (5) providing opportunity for active practice; and (6) providing pleasant learning conditions. Thoughtful planning with these factors in mind helps to maximize any learning experience.

Several methods have been described and evaluated for the teaching of surgical skills and surgical procedures. The lack of uniformity in evaluation and relative lack of comparative data makes it difficult to claim that any method is superior to the others. It is likely that many methods will find a place in surgical teaching, complementing one another to create a more comprehensive training program.

One method of teaching surgical skills is the surgical video. This allows the learner to observe a procedure before entering the operating room or to review it afterward. The obvious advantages include convenience and ease of use, little expenditure of resources, and the ability to view the procedure, in whole or in part, multiple times. It also provides the inexperienced resident with a better view than he or she often gets as a second assistant and with the added luxury of being able to reach for a textbook. The primary drawback of this learning modality is the lack of interaction. Vikram and colleagues [10] sought to overcome this negative quality by creating a computer-based CD-ROM program with video images of a vaginal hysterectomy that fade into three-dimensional schematics and interactive question and answer sessions. Both residents and students perceived this instructional method positively and most rated it as more valuable than direct observation in the operating room.

Beyond observation and knowledge of the steps of a surgical procedure, training requires acquisition of the fundamental physical skills inherent in surgery. Desire for high fidelity or realistic simulation in surgical skills training has led to use of animal models. Animals or cadavers and inanimate models have been used effectively [11–13]. The use of cadavers or animal laboratories may be impractical in many settings for reasons ranging from unavailability of space or animals to the costs being prohibitive. To this end, when comparing a low-fidelity (silicone tubing) model with a high-fidelity model (live rat vas deferens) for teaching microsurgical skills, Grober and coworkers [12] found that the groups fared similarly by most outcome measures, with the low-fidelity model being much less expensive.

Virtual reality simulations represent another nontissue method of teaching basic and advanced surgical skills, having the added benefit of being reusable. These virtual reality trainers have been studied by several groups and found to produce greater skill because more repetitions are performed [14] and lead to increased skill and decreased errors in the operating room compared with controls [15,16]. The use of virtual reality technology is limited by expense, so attention has focused on the less costly approach of laparoscopic video box trainers. The performance of various laparoscopic tasks has been shown to increase trainees' scores on a structured assessment of performance in the surgical theater and in the laboratory setting compared with controls [17,18].

From these results, it is apparent that several specific interventions designed to improve surgical skills are effective in the short term. What has not been addressed is the effectiveness of a structured program incorporating several of these modalities. The combination of a pelvic trainer and animal laboratory has been shown to lead to improved laparoscopic performance for all levels of obstetrics and gynecology residents [13]. A group of general surgery residents evaluated a week-long workshop that included use of lectures, surgical videos, suture boards, interactive teaching sessions, animal laboratories, and virtual reality simulators. The learners were excused from clinical duties for this 5-day period. Although no objective test of performance was administered, the participants consistently found the workshop to be helpful both cognitively and technically [19]. More work needs to be done to answer the question of how best to combine these various instructional techniques, preferably using more objective outcome measures. Designing a precise curriculum based on the needs and resources of a given training program is largely individualized, with the option of incorporating any or all of the proved techniques available.

In light of the promising short-term results, it is important to look at whether these interventions produce any enduring benefits. One such study compared residents who had completed a 2-year curriculum in a surgical skills center with a control group without the additional training. The evaluation instrument was an Objective Structured Assessment of Surgical Skills (OSATS). The intervention group fared no better on the OSATS in their third year of residency than the control group. The trainees, however, did subjectively believe that the program was valuable [20]. Despite this discouraging finding, it would be interesting to know whether the established immediate benefits of the interventions translate into improvements in patient safety, operating time, and costs, especially in the early period of a resident's surgical experience. To assess this question, a retrospective cohort study of laparoscopic outcomes showed operative time, blood loss, hospital stay, and conversion to laparotomy were less frequent for a group of residents that had undergone a formal laparoscopic training program consisting of didactics, bench exercises, instrumentation instruction, animate tissue model surgery, and supervised gynecologic operating experience [21].

Naturally, for both its learning and service-oriented value, operating room experience in real time continues to be a large and important part of surgical training. In an ideal world, it might seem wise for these to happen in sequence, with the high-stakes operating room experience being reserved for the trainee who has mastered the basic technical skills in the laboratory. This approach is not possible in many circumstances. Some basic skills should definitely be taught before any operating room experience, but the integration of laboratory-based training has to happen, in part, concomitantly with the operating room experience. It continues to be the responsibility of the attending physician to ensure patient safety, while allowing for resident participation at an appropriate level. One benefit of laboratory-based teaching and evaluation may be the ability to glean a more objective view of the appropriate level of participation in live surgery for a given surgical trainee.

Selecting evaluation strategies

Within a curriculum, the benchmark or standard for achieving an educational goal helps determine the assessment method. Although there are many different

---

Box 2. Evaluation methods for surgical technical skills

- Examinations, oral or written
- Review of procedure or case logs
- Review of morbidity and mortality data
- Direct observation and assessment
- Direct observation with evaluation criteria
- Performance on animate or bench models
- Review of videotaped performance
- Skills checklists
- Global rating forms
- Virtual reality simulators

---

performance assessment methods available (Box 2), any evaluation strategy should be feasible, reliable, and valid.

Choosing an evaluation strategy depends on several important factors. Issues of assessment reliability and validity must be weighed against factors, such as costs (monetary, time, space, and personnel) and availability of a given evaluation method. Traditional, subjective evaluation by attending physicians, often remote from any meaningful interaction with the resident, is still the norm within most residency programs [22]. This is true despite a significant accumulation of evidence that this type of evaluation is unreliable [4,23]. More than one evaluation method can be applied to technical skills performance, as seen with the OSATS instrument [24]. Numerous studies in the gynecology and general surgery literature have evaluated these more structured and objective methods of assessing performance with good results. Many of these methods of evaluation have been shown to have high construct validity, reliability, and interrater reliability [24–31]. These same strong psychometric properties were seen with the OSATS when the participants were assessed by both blinded and unblinded evaluators [26]. Similar validated measures of performance should be adopted as an integral part of any well-designed curriculum. Actual choice of an evaluation strategy is based on overall resources and the outcomes-related stakes.

Organizing an implementation plan

Managing the many components and details that comprise a surgical skills curriculum is one key to its successful realization. An effective approach to this otherwise daunting task is to formulate a curriculum management plan. Such a document accomplishes several important things: (1) identifies component tasks and the necessary resources for each part of the curriculum; (2) elaborates responsibilities for the stakeholders; and (3) provides timelines for development, implementation, and evaluation of the curriculum. In effect, the curriculum management plan becomes the working charter for those responsible for developing, administering, teaching, and evaluating the curriculum.

When developing a management plan, a surprising amount of detail emanates from a global curricular concept or goal. Without a management plan, details may be overlooked, threatening the overall success of the effort. The following are examples of the types of questions that are often overlooked until the management plan is detailed:

- How will residents receive information and be oriented to the course?
- Who will procure the teaching materials and arrange resource provision?
- How will the curriculum time relate to competing residency activities?
- Who will conduct the necessary faculty development?
- By what process will the curriculum be evaluated and revised?

By anticipating the details, accommodations can be built into the curriculum management plan prospectively, providing a sounder basis for resource allocation.

Imbedded in any implementation plan should be a mechanism for regularly evaluating and revising a curriculum. Once the program is in place and being used, it is necessary to evaluate the effectiveness of the program. Depending on the goals of the program, the depth to which the program is evaluated varies, and there is some dependence on the published data from other institutions to ensure that a valid program is being administered. Part of the evaluation consists of testing the participants in the program, comparing individuals' precourse and postcourse scores on various components of the OSATS. It is also likely that the curriculum administrator will seek subjective feedback from the trainees, their assessment of how educational and user-friendly is the program, and suggestions for improvement. Feedback has to be reviewed periodically, keeping in mind the changing needs of surgical training and continuously updating the program. As technology changes and new evidence continues to mount in both the clinical and educational literature, the program is never finished; rather, it continues as a work in progress. The curriculum management plan serves as a guide for this ongoing monitoring and improvement.

Implementation of a surgical skills curriculum is essentially the culmination of all the preceding steps. Success depends on a well-conceived curriculum management plan and a readiness to be flexible when executing the curriculum, because unforeseen circumstances often necessitate modification of the plan. Similar to the curriculum management plan, an implementation checklist, delineating tasks, the responsible agent, and completion due dates for each component task can also be helpful for curriculum implementation. Actualizing even a small curricular project involves many details. The more time and effort invested in the organization of the curriculum, the greater the chances of successful implementation.

Every curriculum has its strengths and weaknesses and inevitably problems arise. Realistically, no project manager can predict and plan for all contingencies.

Knowing what pitfalls are common may help to avoid them. Examples of such problems include

1. Incompletely planning a curriculum
2. Presenting too much information or instructional content for the time allowed
3. Failing to focus the content and educational objectives
4. Providing too few or poorly choosing faculty for a given instructional exercise
5. Neglecting adequate faculty development

Implementation represents a very large effort best affected by a stepwise and team approach.

Summary

Considerable change is underway in surgical education. Learning the technical elements of surgery, once the by-product of apprenticeship level experience, is now the focus of discussion among residents, educators, accreditation body administrators, patients, and the public. They are all stakeholders in the important task of how future surgeons are trained. An outcomes-based approach to surgical training seems in principle to satisfy best the need for public accountability and patient safety in surgical education. To achieve the goal of developing surgical competence in definable, reliable, and valid outcomes measures, well-designed, coherent technical skills training curricula are necessary. Surgical educators need to understand the basic principles of curriculum design and be willing to apply these educational methods. Beginning with the education goals in mind, curriculum development is attainable when the model is systematically applied and appropriately detailed. In turn, residents, teachers, and patients all are beneficiaries in the process.

References

[1] Patil NG, Cheng SWK, Wong J. Surgical competence. World J Surg 2003;27:943–7.
[2] Cuschieri A, Francis N, Crosby J, et al. What do master surgeons think of surgical competence and revalidation? Am J Surg 2001;182:110–6.
[3] Satava RM, Gallagher AG, Pellegrini CA. Surgical competence and surgical proficiency: definitions, taxonomy, and metrics. J Am Coll Surg 2003;196:933–7.
[4] Reznick RK. Teaching and testing technical skills. Am J Surg 1993;165:358–61.
[5] Accreditation Council for Graduate Medical Education Outcomes Project. Available at: http://www.acgme.org/outcome/project/proHome.asp. Accessed September 1, 2005.
[6] Ritchie Jr WP. The measurement of competence: current plans and future initiatives of the American Board of Surgery. Bull Am Coll Surg 2001;86:10–5.

[7] Gallagher AG, Ritter EM, Champion H, et al. Virtual reality simulation for the operating room: proficiency-based training as a paradigm shift in surgical skills training. Ann Surg 2005; 241:364–72.

[8] Smith JB, Lee VE, Newmann FM. Instruction and achievement in Chicago elementary schools: improving Chicago's schools. Chicago: Consortium on Chicago School Research; 2001.

[9] DesCoteaux J, Leclere H. Learning surgical technical skills. Can J Surg 1995;38:33–8.

[10] Vikram J, Widdowson S, Duffy S. Development and evaluation of an interactive computer-assisted learning program: a novel approach to teaching gynaecological surgery. Br J Educ Technol 2002;33:323–31.

[11] Goff BA, Lentz GM, Lee DM, et al. Formal teaching of surgical skills in an obstetric-gynecologic residency. Obstet Gynecol 1999;93:785–90.

[12] Grober ED, Hamstra SJ, Wanzel KR, et al. The educational impact of bench model fidelity on the acquisition of technical skill: the use of clinically relevant outcome measures. Ann Surg 2004; 240:374–81.

[13] Cundiff GW. Analysis of the effectiveness of an endoscopy education program in improving residents' laparoscopic skills. Obstet Gynecol 1997;90:854–9.

[14] Brunner WC, Korndorffer JR, Sierra R, et al. Laparoscopic virtual reality training: are 30 repetitions enough? J Surg Res 2004;122:150–6.

[15] Grantcharov TP, Kristiansen VB, Bendix J, et al. Randomized clinical trial of virtual reality simulation for laparoscopic skills training. Br J Surg 2004;91:146–50.

[16] Wilhelm DM, Ogan K, Roehrborn CG, et al. Assessment of basic endoscopic performance using a virtual reality simulator. J Am Coll Surg 2002;195:675–81.

[17] Coleman RL, Muller CY. Effects of a laboratory-based skills curriculum on laparoscopic proficiency: a randomized trial. Am J Obstet Gynecol 2002;186:836–42.

[18] Scott DJ, Bergen PC, Rege RV, et al. Laparoscopic training on bench models: better and more cost effective than operating room experience? J Am Coll Surg 2000;191:272–83.

[19] Heppell J, Beauchamp G, Chollet A. Ten-year experience with a basic technical skills and perioperative management workshop for first-year residents. Can J Surg 1995;38:27–32.

[20] Anastakis DJ, Wanzel KR, Brown MH, et al. Evaluating the effectiveness of a 2-year curriculum in a surgical skills center. Am J Surg 2003;185:378–85.

[21] Whitted RW, Pietro PA, Martin G, et al. A retrospective study evaluating the impact of formal laparoscopic training on patient outcomes in a residency program. J Am Assoc Gynecol Laparosc 2003;10:484–8.

[22] Mandel LP, Lentz GM, Goff BA. Teaching and evaluating surgical skills. Obstet Gynecol 2000; 95:783–5.

[23] Watts J, Feldman WB. Assessment of technical skills (assessing clinical competence). New York: Springer; 1985.

[24] Martin JA, Regehr G, Reznick R, et al. Objective structured assessment of technical skill (OSATS) for surgical residents. Br J Surg 1997;84:273–8.

[25] Winckel CP, Reznick RK, Cohen R, et al. Reliability and construct validity of a structured technical skills assessment form. Am J Surg 1994;167:423–7.

[26] Goff BA, Nielsen PE, Lentz GM, et al. Surgical skills assessment: a blinded examination of obstetrics and gynecology residents. Am J Obstet Gynecol 2002;186:613–7.

[27] Goff BA, Lentz GM, Lee D, et al. Development of a bench station objective structured assessment of technical skills. Obstet Gynecol 2001;98:412–6.

[28] Lentz GM, Mandel LS, Lee D, et al. Testing surgical skills of obstetric and gynecologic residents in a bench laboratory setting: validity and reliability. Am J Obstet Gynecol 2001;184:1462–70.

[29] Goff BA, Lentz GM, Lee D, et al. Development of an objective structured assessment of technical skills for obstetric and gynecology residents. Obstet Gynecol 2000;96:46–50.

[30] Reznick R, Regehr G, MacRae H, et al. Testing technical skill via an innovative "bench station" examination. Am J Surg 1996;172:226–30.

[31] Derossis AM, Fried GM, Abrahamowicz M, et al. Development of a model for training and evaluation of laparoscopic skills. Am J Surg 1998;175:482–7.

ELSEVIER
SAUNDERS

Obstet Gynecol Clin N Am
33 (2006) 259–265

OBSTETRICS AND
GYNECOLOGY
CLINICS
OF NORTH AMERICA

The Objective Structured Assessment of Technical Skills and the ACGME Competencies

Carmen J. Sultana, MD

Department of Obstetrics and Gynecology, Jefferson Medical College, 834 Chestnut Street, Suite 400, Philadelphia, PA 19107, USA

Assessment drives both how a subject is taught and what is taught. The Accreditation Council for Graduate Medical Education (ACGME) Outcomes Project has provided a new impetus for residency training programs to examine and improve the way in which they teach technical skills to residents and assess the acquisition of those skills. Pressure from hospitals and other organizations on residency programs to credential residents in specific procedures has emerged as another factor driving change in both surgical teaching and evaluation. The ACGME mandate to assess competency (in this case, surgical skills falls under patient care and medical knowledge) means that programs are looking for tools with which to measure the technical skills of their residents. The Objective Structured Assessment of Technical Skills (OSAT) is a variation on the Objective Structured Clinical Examination. It is one of the newer tools used to assess competency. The OSAT is cited in the ACGME Evaluation Toolbox on their website as the most desirable evaluation tool for the patient care topics including interviewing, counseling, preventive services, and performance of physical examinations. Simulators and models are listed as most desirable tools for evaluating medical procedures. An OSAT combines both evaluation of patient care topics and evaluation of medical procedures. This article reviews the history of teaching technical skills, components of surgical skills assessment, definition of an OSAT, and suggestions for future development of surgical skills assessment tools.

E-mail address: carmen.sultana@jefferson.edu

Why evaluate or teach outside the operating room setting? Until recently, the cognitive apprenticeship model of learning, in which residents learned by working side by side with experienced surgeons in a real life setting, was the major method with which to impart surgical skills. The framework for this transformation of novice to expert exploits several components. It relies on role modeling and relationships with the instructor who coaches the learner. A scaffolding or framework of basic skills is built on as learners articulate or string together the steps of the procedures being taught, eventually acquiring the ability to perform progressively more complex procedures. The apprentice model is limited by the availability of mentors and their teaching ability, the variable types of procedures and patients that are available for training, and the important issues of how to maintain patient safety and the quality of care while attending to the needs of the learner.

Reznick [1], whose group has many publications on the subject of teaching and evaluating surgical skills, noted that the "Most important ingredient (of surgical teaching) is the appreciation of the importance of ... skill acquisition accompanied by the access to a knowledgeable patient faculty." He cites the importance of perception, integration, and automatization [2]. Perception is the awareness of the essentials of procedures, integration refers to learning of the framework and steps, and automatization occurs after repetition. In addition to these concepts, those teaching residents should also be aware of the ways in which adults learn. Adults set goals and objectives for skills they wish to acquire, which affects their interest in a given subject. They tend to focus on tasks rather than on abstract knowledge. They also display metacognition, or an awareness of their own learning strategies and preferences. In keeping with this, the instructor of adult learners needs to be centered on the learner rather than solely on the subject material. He or she should assess the learner's level of skill brought to the situation so that the new knowledge can be integrated with knowledge or skills previously learned. Transferable concepts should be emphasized. Formative evaluation, or ongoing feedback to the learner, is also important.

In creating a new approach to surgical assessment, three components should be addressed: (1) feasibility, (2) reliability, and (3) validity. Evaluation methods that are feasible can be done easily and inexpensively. Reliable methods are reproducible and precise. Validity can be thought of as "are we measuring what we intend to"? A valid test is predictive, or forecasts future performance and has appropriate content, which for the assessment of surgical skills means that it would measure technical skill rather than medical knowledge. In addition, a valid test is concurrent if it correlates with some gold standard, and has construct validity or the ability to separate groups. Finally, a valid test must have face validity or resemble the real world.

How can one incorporate this information into the development of an assessment method? Commonly used global rating forms do not accurately discriminate skills and are ranked low in preferred methods by the ACGME. Watts and Feldman [3] evaluated procedure logs, direct observation, direct observation with criteria, animal models with criteria, and videotapes in terms of reliability and validity. They gave the highest rating to direct observation with criteria, noting that the performance of models and videotaping depended on the degree of realism achieved.

One method of direct observation with criteria is the Global Rating Scale of Operative Performance that is part of the ACGME Toolbox (Fig. 1) [4]. The components assessed include respect for tissues, time and motion, instrument handling, knowledge of instruments, flow of the operation, uses of assistants, and knowledge of specific procedure on a five-point Likert scale. The same author went on to develop a structured technical skills assessment form that partitioned particular procedures into their smallest fundamental components [5]. This was done for cholecystectomy, hernia repair, and bowel repair. It included a 10-point summary scale; had high levels of interrater reliability; and was able to differentiate junior from senior residents, suggesting construct validity.

The logical next step for investigators was to control the assessment environment by doing structured evaluations in a bench setting with models instead of in the operating room. An initial trial in 1996 used eight 15-minute bench stations for simulated skin excision, T-tube insertion, abdominal wall closure, bowel anastomosis, inferior vena cava hemorrhage, pyloroplasty, and tracheostomy [4]. The exercise required 48 surgeon examiners to spend 2 hours each to examine all their residents, with a cost of about $200 Canadian per resident. They established an interstation reliability of 0.843 for the global rating and 0.781 for the checklist. ANOVA showed a significant difference according to training level, implying construct validity.

The same group of investigators then set out to compare the use of live animals with the bench models [6]. Again, they used 48 examiners who spent 3 hours each to examine 20 residents, using six stations. All residents went through both types of stations. Three ratings methods were used: (1) checklists, (2) global rating forms, and (3) pass-fail judgments. The ANOVA results showed that the scores for the two examiners correlated for all three methods. The reliability indices for the checklist and global scores were moderate to high. Internal consistency was moderate to high for the live checklist. Both formats were equivalent for the global rating. The global rating was better at differentiating resident levels. They noted that they need more stations to have higher reliability. The conclusion was that the bench models were equivalent to the use of anesthetized animals, at a cost of $160 versus $600. In another study, the same authors compared bench models with cadavers and textbook training in six procedures using the same checklists and global rating scales and found that cadaver and bench models were superior to textbook teaching [7].

Other investigators have similar findings in an obstetrics and gynecology program. Goff and coworkers [8] described pig laboratory teaching sessions on knot tying, suturing, tying on a passer, laparoscopic tasks using pegs, and transferring objects from one instrument to another. The animal laboratories included tubal ligation, ostomy, salpingectomy, open repair of cystotomy, enterotomy, salpingo-oophorectomy, hypogastric artery ligation, and more advanced procedures. A written pretest and posttest 6 months later was used. The subjec-

GLOBAL RATING SCALE OF OPERATIVE PERFORMANCE

Please circle the number corresponding to the candidate's performance in each category, irrespective of training level.

Respect for Tissue:

1	2	3	4	5
Frequently used unnecessary force on tissue or caused damage by inappropriate use of instruments		Careful handling of tissue but occasionally caused inadvertent damage		Consistently handled tissues appropriately with minimal damage

Time and Motion:

1	2	3	4	5
Many unnecessary moves		Efficient time/motion but some unnecessary moves		Clear economy of movement and maximum efficiency

Instrument Handling:

1	2	3	4	5
Repeatedly makes tentative or awkward moves with instruments by inappropriate use of instruments		Competent use of instruments but occasionally appeared stiff or awkward		Fluid moves with instruments and no awkwardness

Knowledge of Instrument:

1	2	3	4	5
Frequently asked for wrong instrument or used inappropriate instrument		Knew names of most instruments and used appropriate instrument		Obviously familiar with the instruments and their names

Flow of Operation:

1	2	3	4	5
Frequently stopped operating and seemed unsure of next move		Demonstrated some forward planning with reasonable progression of procedure		Obviously planned course of operation with effortless flow from one move to the next

Use of Assistants:

1	2	3	4	5
Consistently placed assistants poorly or failed to use assistants		Appropriate use of assistants most of the time		Strategically used assistants to the best advantage at all times

Knowlegde of Specific Procedure:

1	2	3	4	5
Deficient knowledge. Needed specific instruction at most steps		Knew all important steps of operation		Demonstrated familiarity with all aspects of operation

OVERALL ON THIS TASK, SHOULD THE CANDIDATE: FAIL   PASS

tive faculty evaluation differentiated resident training levels and residents believed the laboratories improved their skills. Subsequent studies included a seven-station, 4-hour, $1500 pig laboratory. The procedure included laparoscopic port placement, salpingostomy, suturing, vessel ligation and open hypogastric artery ligation, enterotomy repair, and salpingo-oophorectomy. Residents were evaluated with a task-specific checklist, global rating scale, and pass-fail grade. They also used self-scored and skills ratings by the faculty [9]. The reliability and construct validity of the evaluations were high. The next two studies by this group used bench models instead of live animals. Lentz and coworkers [10] used a written test and 12 stations including six laparoscopic procedures, four abdominal, and a knot tying station at a cost of $50 each. The residents were scored on time and a five-point scale by two examiners. The results showed that the global ratings performed better than the checklists. Reliability varied with the task, but overall was 0.79. The construct validity was best with the total score.

This group later repeated this study in a blinded fashion with seven stations, and found similar results for construct validity and reliability [11]. One examiner of an examiner pair for each resident did not know the resident. The feasibility of this evaluation instrument was further examined by administering a version of their OSAT examination to a total of 116 residents from five different programs [12]. One of the programs was the site where they had performed the original exercises in teaching and evaluation. The combination of one blinded and one unblinded examiner was again used, with an overall interrater reliability of 0.95 (range, 0.71–0.97). The test consisted of three open and three laparoscopic tasks, and took each resident 90 minutes. Both the global rating and checklists discriminated between resident levels. The equipment costs were between $40 and $150 per resident depending on the tasks chosen. Residents who had experienced the groups' laboratory-based curriculum performed better in terms of scores and time to complete tasks than those who were naive to the laboratory setup.

Other trials are few. Coleman and Muller [13] conducted a randomized trial of videotaped laparoscopic salpingectomy after intensive video skills training and noted improvement in timed drill scores in the drill versus control group. Reliability and validity were established for an OSAT for episiotomy repair that evaluated six components of the repair and seven global surgical skills and a pass-fail assessment [14].

In addition to global evaluations and checklists, dexterity analysis systems may in the future provide another level of evaluation [15]. One example, the Isotrack (Polhemus Inc., Colchester, Vermont), is an electromagnetic field generator with sensors that attach to the surgeon's hands and collect information on

Fig. 1. Global rating scale of operative performance. (*From* Reznick RK, Regehr G, MacRae H, et al. Testing technical skill via an innovative bench station examination. Am J Surg 1996;172: 226–30; with permission.)

time and hand movements in performing tasks. Construct validity of this system has been demonstrated, and it has been used in assessment of laparoscopic and open tasks [16,17]. Virtual reality systems, such as the MIST-VR minimally invasive surgical trainer, were developed through a task analysis of a surgical procedure, then replicated in the virtual domain. Metrics, such as economy of movement, length of path, and instrument errors, have been used to validate the assessment of basic laparoscopic skills [18,19].

Bench models for testing surgical skills seem to be effective tools for identifying and differentiating levels of resident skills at an inexpensive cost. Many examples of specific models are in the literature or presented at meetings. The evaluation can be incorporated into a surgical curriculum that programs can tailor to their own needs. Resources include the ACGME Outcomes Project link at www.acgme.org and the Council for Resident Education in Obstetrics and Gynecology (CREOG) Educational Objectives and Surgical Curriculum, via www.acog.org.

References

[1] Reznick RK. Teaching and testing technical skills. Am J Surg 1993;165:358–61.

[2] Kopta JA. An approach to the evaluation of operative skills. Surgery 1971;70:297–303.

[3] Watts J, Feldman WB. Assessment of technical skills. In: Neufeld VR, Norman GR, editors. Assessing clinical competence. New York: Springer; 1985. p. 259–74.

[4] Reznick RK, Regehr G, MacRae H, et al. Testing technical skill via an innovative "bench station" examination. Am J Surg 1996;172:226–30.

[5] Winckel CP, Reznick RK, Cohen R, et al. Reliability and construct validity of a structured technical skills assessment form. Am J Surg 1994;167:423–7.

[6] Martin JA, Regehr G, Reznick RK, et al. Objective structured assessment of technical skill (OSATS) for surgical residents. Br J Surg 1997;84:273–8.

[7] Anastakis D, Regehr G, Reznick RK, et al. Assessment of technical skills transfer from the bench training model to the human model. Am J Surg 1999;177:167–70.

[8] Goff BA, Lentz GM, Lee DM, et al. Formal teaching of surgical skills in an obstetric-gynecologic residency. Obstet Gynecol 1999;93:785–90.

[9] Goff BA, Lentz GM, Lee DM, et al. Development of an objective structured assessment of technical skills for obstetric and gynecology residents. Obstet Gynecol 2000;96:146–50.

[10] Lentz GM, Mandel LS, Lee DM, et al. Testing surgical skills of obstetric and gynecologic residents in a bench laboratory setting: validity and reliability. Am J Obstet Gynecol 2001; 184:1462–70.

[11] Goff BA, Nielson PE, Lentz GM, et al. Surgical skills assessment : a blinded examination of obstetrics and gynecology residents. Am J Obstet Gynecol 2002;186:613–7.

[12] Goff B, Mandel L, Lentz G, et al. Assessment of resident surgical skills: is testing feasible? Am J Obstet Gynecol 2005;192:1331–40.

[13] Coleman RL, Muller CY. Effects of a laboratory-based skills curriculum on laparoscopic proficiency: a randomized trial. Am J Obstet Gynecol 2002;186:836–42.

[14] Nielsen PE, Foglia LM, Mandel LS, et al. Objective structured assessment of technical skills for episiotomy repair. Am J Obstet Gynecol 2003;189:1257–60.

[15] Moorthy K, Munz Y, Sarker SK, et al. Objective assessment of technical skills in surgery. BMJ 2003;327:1032–7.

[16] Datta V, Mackay S, Mandalia M, et al. The use of electromagnetic motion tracking analysis

to objectively measure open surgical skill in the laboratory-based model. J Am Coll Surg 2001;193:479–85.

[17] Mackay S, Datta V, Chang A, et al. Multiple objective measures of skill (MOMS): a new approach to the assessment of technical ability in surgical trainees. Ann Surg 2003;238:291–300.

[18] Taffinder N, Sutton C, Fishwick RJ, et al. Validation of virtual reality to teach and assess psychomotor skills in laparoscopic surgery: results from randomized controlled studies using the MIST-VR laparoscopic simulator. Stud Health Technol Inform 1998;50:124–30.

[19] Bann S, Kwok KF, Lo CY, et al. Objective assessment of technical skills of surgical trainees in Hong Kong. Br J Surg 2003;90:1294–9.

**ELSEVIER
SAUNDERS**

Obstet Gynecol Clin N Am
33 (2006) 267–281

**OBSTETRICS AND
GYNECOLOGY
CLINICS
OF NORTH AMERICA**

From the Simple to the Sublime: Incorporating Surgical Models into Your Surgical Curriculum

Patrick J. Woodman, DO[a,b,c,*], Charles W. Nager, MD[d]

[a]*Department of Obstetrics and Gynecology, University of Indiana School of Medicine,
1120 South Drive, Fesler Hall 302, Indianapolis, IN 46202-5114, USA*
[b]*University of California–San Diego School of Medicine, 9500 Gilman Drive,
La Jolla, CA 92093, USA*
[c]*Urogynecology Associates, 1633 North Capitol Avenue, Indianapolis, IN 46202, USA*
[d]*Division of Urogynecology, Department of Reproductive Medicine,
University of California–San Diego Medical Center, 9350 Campus Point Drive, Suite 2A,
La Jolla, CA 92037–0674, USA*

The early practice of medical training involved a formal apprenticeship with an established physician, typically for a number of years [1]. In the late 1800s, education shifted to university-based medical schools, where one-on-one teaching was replaced by teaching in the classroom [2]. Surgery was observed in theaters, and the resident was given increasing levels of responsibility until he or she could earn the right to assist the surgical attending. In many cases, the first time a surgical trainee performed a complete surgical procedure was after graduation.

In present-day surgical training, an attending physician typically works with one or two assistants, allowing each to do a portion of the surgery commensurate with the residents' experience. This allows the resident more surgical freedom, but it also allows the attending physician to supervise and monitor surgical progress directly. Despite this shift in philosophy, several factors have negatively impacted the quality of graduating physicians.

The Centers for Medicare and Medicaid Services, formally the Health Care Financing Administration, created rules that now require attending physicians

* Corresponding author. Urogynecology Associates, 1633 North Capitol Avenue, Indianapolis, IN 46202.

E-mail address: patrick.woodman@gmail.com (P.J. Woodman).

0889-8545/06/$ – see front matter © 2006 Elsevier Inc. All rights reserved.
doi:10.1016/j.ogc.2006.01.008   *obgyn.theclinics.com*

to examine independently patients treated by trainees [3], adding inefficiency into busy schedules and lowering the number of patients that can be seen. With a renaissance of medical and conservative therapies, fewer surgical procedures are being done, further limiting trainee experience. The recently adopted 80-hour work-week policy may cause surgical specialty residents to miss even more cases [4].

To their benefit, trainees work with a larger number of attending physicians today than they did in the past. This dilutes the exposure attending physicians have with any one trainee, however, making objective evaluation of their performance difficult. More importantly, the medicolegal environment in the United States has indelibly changed the doctor-patient relationship. Patients unrealistically expect surgical perfection without practice. Didactic lectures, reading articles and texts, and surgical assistance are a good foundation for the surgical trainee, but at some point, the trainee performs his or her first case.

It behooves the attending physician to prepare the trainee before entering the operating room. There are several ways to practice surgical skills without live, human subjects. Cadaveric specimens most closely represent live subjects, but are dependent on an available willed-body program. Costs to purchase a cadaver can be prohibitive, and range from $500 to $1500 per body. An appropriate morgue must have space for the cadavers, and there may be heated competition to use the specimens if the institution has several training programs. Embalmed cadavers are subject to rigor mortis, which limits their usefulness for practicing surgical technique. Unembalmed cadavers have limited longevity. In addition, cadavers have no dynamic muscle tone, leading to distortions in anatomy. Finally, cadavers lead to a false sense of security because surgery on a cadaver produces no bleeding.

Animal models are wonderful alternatives to human experimentation and overcome some of the previously mentioned limitations. In many cases, animal models are limited because the chosen animal anatomy may not accurately represent human anatomy. Tissues and organs tend to be smaller than the human analog, and the resident trainee might benefit from a slightly bigger specimen. Purchase of animals is cheaper than human cadavers; however, live animal experiments may involve the care and feeding of those animals, which adds to their cost. Animal laboratory costs can be prohibitive, and run about $450 per square foot, depending on space efficiency [5]. Legal restrictions limit what can be done with animal subjects and private groups, such as People for the Ethical Treatment of Animals, also oppose the use of animals in surgical training.

Inanimate models

Inanimate models are three-dimensional representations of an anatomic specimen, a surgical procedure, or a process. They mimic the visual-spatial relationships that are difficult to conceptualize from reading a journal or text, or looking at a photograph. It allows the trainee to practice the hand-eye coordination necessary to perform a surgical task. After an initial outlay of capital funds, many models are reusable, or the model components can be made from commonly available materials.

Models' cost can range from a few pennies to thousands of dollars. As the complexity or the realism of the model increases, so does the cost. Other drawbacks include the inanimate nature of most models that limits the learning of the dynamic properties and interactions the trainee encounters with a living patient. Developers of a model typically try to imitate reality by asking the trainee to perform an analogous task, which may or may not approximate reality when performing the mimicked task. Models cannot reproduce all the complex processes needed to perform surgery on a living human being.

The surgeon, when performing an operation, focuses on a particular task or goal (ie, the removal of a diseased organ), but models can emphasize certain component steps. The resident trainee can focus on difficult portions of the procedure, before they perform the procedure on a patient. This practice comes without risk to the patient.

Models can be used to teach basic skills that all surgeons should know. For instance, all surgeons tie surgical knots and the "knot board" can be something as simple as a plank of wood with a hook attached, used as a platform on which the trainee can tie suture [6]. Wound closure models can be a simple sheet of wool felt that the trainee is asked to sew into a tube, a pig's foot that the trainee slices and repairs [7], or as complex as silicone tissue (Wound Closure model, Surgical Training Aids, Hollywood, South Carolina), with or without a mechanism to pump artificial blood. Although a surgeon closes thousands of lacerations or incisions in his or her career, practice before the first repair can theoretically improve results, decrease surgical time, and offers the trainee a safe environment to make mistakes.

Repetition is key. Every procedure, no matter how simple, has a learning curve. When certain aspects of a procedure become automatic, then complications drop exponentially [8]. An example comes from Shouldice Hospital, a hernia hospital outside Toronto, Canada. Most experienced surgeons have an inguinal hernia failure rate of between 10% and 15%. In the Shouldice experience, without the use of synthetic meshes, their failure rate is 1%. How do the surgeons explain their superb success rate? The surgeons at Shouldice do between 6000 and 8000 hernia operations per year, more than most surgeons do in a lifetime. With repetition, they make complex moves and decisions automatically [9]. Practice can make perfect (or rather, nearly).

Models allow one instructor to teach several students at once. Each can watch their colleagues use the model, before they try themselves. This allows both conceptual and visual learners to benefit [10]. Movements can be practiced again and again until they are automatic. Most resident trainees only perform 500 to 1000 major surgeries during training [11], so they do not have time in the operating room to waste learning to tie knots.

As the trainee progresses from simple to more complicated procedures, models can be an after-hours platform for practice. Success at endoscopic procedures, such as laparoscopy, cystoscopy, and hysteroscopy, depends a great deal on familiarity with the equipment and hand-eye coordination with the instruments, constrained by the soft tissue of entry ports. It is difficult to adjust seeing the surgical landscape in two dimensions when one has only experienced it in three.

The clinical finding of breast cancer underlines the use of models to practice rare procedures or respond to uncommon complications or findings. Breast examinations are an example. Resident trainees are expected to be experts at detecting lesions and cancer, and are also expected to be able to teach patients to detect their own abnormalities. A breast examination model with several abnormalities (ie, Breast Exam Model, Kappa Medical, Prescott, Arizona) is an excellent tool for both clinician and patient to detect breast lesions.

Another example is the repair of third- and fourth-degree anal sphincter lacerations. In many training programs, obstetrics and gynecology residents may have the opportunity to repair three or four anal sphincter lacerations during their 4-year residency. Nonetheless, the trainee must be prepared and practiced when these severe lacerations occur. Several models have been developed that mimic the steps needed for episiorrhaphy. These models allow the trainee to practice the complicated tasks necessary to repair the defect.

General surgeons may get ample opportunity to treat trauma patients. Trainees in other surgical specialties, like obstetrics and gynecology, may have only a fleeting opportunity to manage trauma, perhaps in a military deployment or during an advanced trauma life support course. TraumaMan HPS (Simulab, Seattle, Washington) provides participants with a chance to place a realistic chest tube, decompress a pneumothorax or a distended pericardium, perform a venous cut-down, or intubate an obtunded patient [12]. The model attendant can mimic the pumping of blood, the breath sounds of the lungs, and a fluid wave of the acute abdomen. To practice running a code, the Human Patient Simulator (Medical Education Technologies, Sarasota, Florida) uses a computer module that allows for interaction with the "patient" and allows the instructor to control the vital signs, the electrocardiogram tracing, oxygen saturation, and responsiveness and allows the trainee to administer medications.

Models can also be used to measure or track trainee performance. If a model is found to have face validity and predictive validity, then the model should be sensitive to change. The Objective Structured Assessment of Technical Skills has been used to objectively rate a trainee's performance on a relatively subjective task [13]. They have been developed for tasks as varied as anesthetic placement to small bowel anastomosis [14–17]. Objective Structured Assessment of Technical Skills can limit the subjective influences of personality, previous performance, age, and gender bias. Documentation of multiple failures on a task provides written evidence of inadequate performance.

The Cumulative Sum Score is a grading system that can be used to track trainee performance at three basic surgical procedures [18]. Minimal standards are set for the amount of time necessary to complete a task, then criteria for a "pass" are established. Adequate performance of the task in a set time frame results in a score of −0.1. Failing the task results in a +0.9 score. Initial Cumulative Sum Score scores are positive during the first part of the learning curve; however, as the trainee improves, the Cumulative Sum Score curve should plateau over time. Ultimately, the trainee has to succeed nine times for every failure. Those trainees with a delay in the plateau can be selected for additional instruction. Those who never plateau can be chosen for remediation or termination.

Technical challenges to model development

From the simplest knot board, to the complicated Human Patient Simulator, many challenges surround the development of a surgical model. The initial task is to design a model that represents the task in question and that allows the learner to reproduce skills needed to complete a surgical task. The choice of materials is not necessarily paramount: if the materials mimic the look and feel of biologic tissue, then so much the better. Many simple models, however, do not have to reproduce, for instance, the look of the inside of the abdomen. The task must simply reproduce the biomechanical properties required to perform the task (ie, go through the motions, the resistance of tissue). An example of this is the laparoscopic pegboard, in which the trainee must put beads into small cups, pass a bead from hand-to-hand, or tie knots laparoscopically [17]: it matters more that the manual dexterity and equipment skills needed for laparoscopic procedures are practiced than the fact the pegboard does not resemble the peritoneal cavity.

How much preparation time does one have? In many cases, the instructor wants something that can be pulled off the shelf and ready to use. If the model uses perishable material (ie, a pig's foot, a cow's tongue) or disposables, however, then construction of the model might be necessary the night before the teaching session.

Money is the next big issue. Models that use everyday items or discarded or unused surgical items are the most economical. Reusable models may require an initial outlay of money, but may be inexpensive in the long run. Computerized or custom-made models tend to be more expensive.

Models do take up space. For some complicated models, such as an endoscopic trainer, a room is needed not only to store the model, the endoscope, the light source, and a television monitor, but also to provide adequate facilities to run workshops. Storage outside the office can be an issue, with the logistical problem of getting the model out of storage in time for a training session.

To use models to evaluate skills, standardized performance goals must be agreed on by the rating faculty. Models cannot be used alone, and one-on-one demonstrations, videos, or written instruction or lectures should precede the task at hand. Each trainee should know against which criteria they are evaluated so that consistent and fair criteria are used to determine performance.

Last, but not least, the model should be interesting and fun. Residents and other trainees have spent years listening to lectures and memorizing facts. If the model does not pique their interest, then they will be less likely to use it.

Examples of surgical models

The number of surgical models that are available or described is staggering. Although this is by no means an exhaustive list, the following are some examples of models made from everyday materials, cost ranging from $2 to $145. These models were submitted by members of the American Urogynecologic Society, and were presented at postgraduate courses at the twenty-fifth and twenty-sixth American Urogynecologic Society Annual Scientific Meetings and a recent Annual Convention of the Association of Professors in Gynecology and Obstetrics/Council on Resident Education in Obstetrics and Gynecology. More models can be accessed

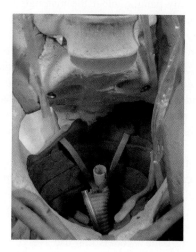

Fig. 1. Materials required for female clay pelvis model. (Courtesy of Myers et al, Providence, RI.)
One model pelvis
One left femur
Modeling clay, four colors
Green cord or white twine (nerves)
Straw (urethra)
Aortic graft (vagina)
Thick rubber band, cut (uterosacral ligaments)
Vinyl tablecloth
Rolling pin
Modeling clay shaping tools
Paper templates of muscle groups
Paper towels
Hemostats
Atlas of human anatomy (ie, Netter)

through these groups' websites: http://www.acog.org/CREOGskills or http://www.acog.org/departments/download/SurgicalCurriculum.pdf.

Female clay pelvis model

Myers and coworkers [19] from Brown University developed an anatomic model of the pelvis that the trainee builds. The concept is to teach the participant clinical anatomy by building it from the bones up. A standard plastic anatomic pelvis and femur is used, with different colors of clay used to represent muscles and ligaments. The model costs approximately $145 and is reusable. The model takes 2 hours to set up, but anatomy is learned during the building process. Each model can be used for two learners and one proctor at a time (Figs. 1 and 2).

Muscle templates are made by tracing muscle groups on paper. Gray clay is used to develop the ligamentous structures of the pelvis and the obturator membrane, and red and orange clay is used for muscles. Muscle groups are built and laid in the pelvis, referring to a course syllabus or the human anatomy text. Analogues for the uterosacral ligament, vagina, rectum, urethra, and nerves are used, until the pelvis is built, excluding subcutaneous tissue and skin.

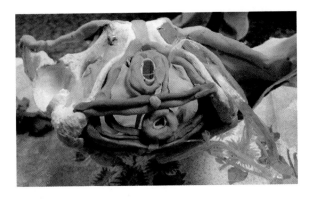

Fig. 2. Materials required for female clay pelvis model. (Courtesy of Myers et al, Providence, RI.)
One model pelvis
One left femur
Modeling clay, four colors
Green cord or white twine (nerves)
Straw (urethra)
Aortic graft (vagina)
Thick rubber band, cut (uterosacral ligaments)
Vinyl tablecloth
Rolling pin
Modeling clay shaping tools
Paper templates of muscle groups
Paper towels
Hemostats
Atlas of human anatomy (ie, Netter)

Sacrocolpopexy

A model for sacrocolpopexy was developed by Rogers at the University of New Mexico, using window screen and a stuffed sock. One of the more difficult parts of the sacrocolpopexy is the placement of suture through the mesh, working with a partner and suture management, all of which this model allows the participant to practice. Preparatory time is about 10 minutes, and the cost for materials is about $2, excluding surgical instruments (Fig. 3).

To begin, a sock is stuffed and the "anterior" and "posterior" sides are marked for the trainee. Two pieces of window screening are prepared using the stuffed sock as a template. This model allows the trainee to begin to understand the requisite motions needed to sew a mesh to the vagina, the importance of exposure, and ways to deal with the difficulty of suture management.

Colpocleisis

Rogers also developed a model for colpocleisis using two socks and a piece of cardboard tubing. The colpocleisis is not technically difficult, but it is hard to conceptually grasp by reading alone. Preparatory time is about 10 minutes, and cost is minimal (Fig. 4).

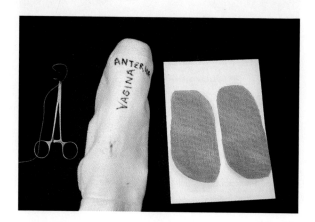

Fig. 3. Materials required for abdominosacral colpopexy model. (Courtesy of Rebecca Rogers, MD, Albuquerque, NM.)
One sock
Suture
Stuffing (ie, rolled newspaper)
Four allis clamps
Needle driver, pick-ups, and scissors
Suture
Two cut pieces window screen (mesh)
Tape and paper
Markers

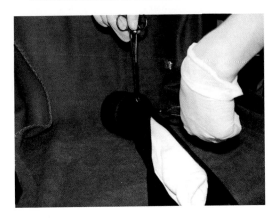

Fig. 4. Materials required for colpocleisis model. (Courtesy of Rebecca Rogers, MD, Albuquerque, NM.)
Two socks
Suture
3–4-in diameter cardboard tubing
Needle driver, pick-ups, and scissors
Four allis clamps
Tape

To begin, place one sock inside the other and secure the open end of the sock over the tube opening with tape. The tube pieces should be cut to a length of approximately 3 in. The trainee can then identify the prolapsed "cuff" (toe of the other sock) and open the "epithelium," eventually trimming the sock approximately 1 to 2 cm from the "introitus" (rubber tube). The adventitia of the vagina (inside sock) can then be imbricated in the fashion of colpocleisis and then the vaginal epithelium closed.

Sacrospinous ligament fixation model

Woodman at Indiana University/Methodist Hospital in Indianapolis developed a sacrospinous ligament fixation model, made from two pieces of plywood, some fabric, a ribbon, and a sock. A participant using this model practices retracting tissue, operating in a deep tube, and penetrating the sacrospinous ligament. Preparatory time is 30 minutes, but the model is reusable. Cost for materials is about $10, excluding surgical instruments (Fig. 5).

To begin, first glue quilt batting to one of the pieces of plywood. When dry, repeat with fabric: this provides a platform for the ribbon and sock to be attached to the model. Hammer the two plywood pieces together in an L- shaped configuration. Take the upholstery tack and screw the tack through the ribbon and toe of the sock onto the fabric-covered piece of plywood. A second upholstery tack anchors the ribbon against the sock and firmly suspends the sock from the board.

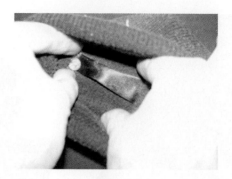

Fig. 5. Materials required for sacrospinous ligament bench model. (Courtesy of Patrick Woodman, DO, Indianapolis, IN.)
One sock (prolapsed vagina)
Two upholstery pins
One 1- or 2-in wide ribbon
Two square feet fabric
Two square feet quilt batting
Two 1-ft square pieces of plywood
Hammer and nails
Glue gun
Four allis clamps
Suture scissors
Light source
Retractors (ie, Breitsky, right-angle)
Choice of needle driver (ie, Capio, Miya hook, Deschamp's)

The open end of the sock represents the open vaginal cuff that is completely prolapsed and the ribbon represents the coccygeus muscle and sacrospinous ligament. The trainee can throw stitches through the sacrospinous ligament while operating in a long tube, practice pulley stitches, and suspend the vaginal cuff to the ligament.

Beef tongue–turkey leg episiotomy repair model

Davis from the National Capitol Consortium at Walter Reed Army Medical Center developed a fourth-degree episiotomy repair model using a beef tongue and a turkey leg. A transverse cut of the beef tongue has a similar density and fiber direction as the cut perineal body. The models cost about $5 a piece, and a single beef tongue and a package of two turkey legs supplies three models. There is a 30 minute preparation time per model (Fig. 6).

To begin, the beef tongue is first cut into sections of 4-in length. The skin of the turkey leg is dissected from the underlying fascia. This skin can be used to represent anal epithelium for the model. Junior residents can use this exercise to develop basic instrumentation skills, and techniques for mobilizing vaginal epithelium. The broad fascial covering of the turkey leg is then dissected from

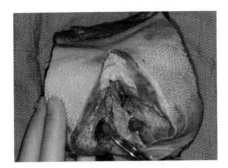

Fig. 6. Materials required for beef tongue–turkey leg model. (Courtesy of Gary Davis, MD, Washington, DC.)
One beef tongue
One turkey leg
Needle drivers, pick-ups, scissors, and scalpel
Suture
Red and blue food coloring

over the muscles. This fascia is used to make a realistic rectovaginal fascia for the model. Just under the broad flat superficial muscle of the turkey leg lie several small round encapsulated muscles with a central tendon, which are dissected free and used to make the external anal sphincter for the model.

An incision is made in the center of the beef tongue section to resemble an obstetric laceration. The section of turkey leg fascia is sutured to the top of the laceration and placed laterally to represent the rectovaginal fascia. The skin from the turkey leg can be sutured to the bottom of the laceration to represent the anal epithelium, and holds sutures much like the actual tissue.

Finally, a hemostat is used to penetrate the lateral sides of the beef tongue section with the points coming out inside the "laceration." The small tendon of the round encapsulated muscles removed from the turkey leg is then grasped and pulled out to the side of the beef tongue section. The muscle and its' capsule resemble a transected external anal sphincter. The key anatomic structures can be colored with cake icing color or any water-color paints for a more realistic effect.

Papier-mâché cystoscopy model

Handa from Johns Hopkins developed a papier-mâché bladder model that can be used to practice cystoscopy. It allows the participant to familiarize themselves with the cystoscopic sheath, bridge, and various cystoscopes and to practice visualization using differently angled endoscopes. The model costs $10, but does take some initial preparatory work (Fig. 7).

The balloon is inflated and then covered with papier-mâché. After drying (usually a few hours), the balloon is removed, the "bladder" is cut in half, and using markers, the trigone is drawn at the bladder base. Unknown "lesions" can

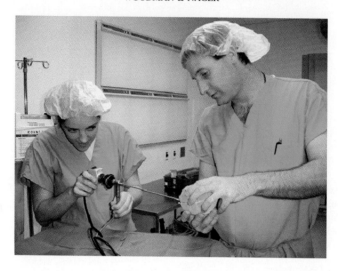

Fig. 7. Materials required for papier-mâché cystoscopy model. (Courtesy of Victoria Handa, MD, Baltimore, MD.)
One balloon / model
Papier-mâché paste
Newspaper
Markers
Tape
Cystoscopic equipment (0-degree, 70-degree rigid endoscopes; sheath; bridges; light source [camera, television monitor optional])

also be drawn on the internal surface for identification by the trainees. The "bladder" is then put back together and cystoscopy is performed through the opening through which the balloon was removed.

Fajita–candy bar episiotomy repair model

Another model used to practice the repair of a third- or fourth-degree perineal laceration was modified from a model used to teach family practice residents their advanced life support in obstetrics by Rogers at the University of New Mexico [20,21]. Cost is minimal at about $2 a model and several trainees can use the same materials during a session. Set up time is also minimal, taking only a few minutes (Fig. 8).

To construct this model, cut the washcloth so there is a diamond-shaped defect in the middle, with apices representing the edges of the cut or torn hymeneal remnants. Markers can be used to draw lines on the washcloth representing the bulbocavernosis and transverse perineal muscles. A candy bar is wrapped with the tube netting and a 2- to 3-cm incision in the midline is made to represent the torn anal mucosa. This wrapped candy bar is placed on a cut piece of the ace

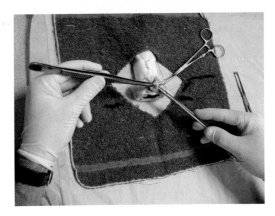

Fig. 8. Materials required for fajita–candy bar episiotomy model. (Courtesy of Rebecca Rogers, MD, Albuquerque, NM.)
One washcloth
One candy bar (anal canal)
One strip flank steak (2 cm × 12 cm)
One needle driver, pick-ups, and scissors
One ace bandage (2 cm × 10 cm)
Two pieces of finger cast netting
Suture
Markers

bandage, representing the torn internal anal sphincter. The remaining piece of the tube netting is placed around the strip of fajita flank steak, representing the torn external anal sphincter inside its fascia. This is placed slightly under the ace bandage: when repaired it lies on top of the repaired "internal anal sphincter."

Watermelon cesarean delivery model

Fenner and Harris from the University of Michigan developed a cesarean delivery model using a watermelon to mimic the gravid abdomen, and various layers of fabric, plastic, and rubber taped to the watermelon to represent the different surgical layers encountered. The model costs only a few dollars, takes 10 minutes to set up, and can be used for two or three learners at a time (Fig. 9).

To begin, fill a balloon with water (to simulate the bladder and urine) and tape it to the lower part of the watermelon, with a double fold at the top to simulate the dome of the bladder. A cardboard toilet-paper roll on top of the bladder simulates the pubic symphysis. Then, lay a piece of plastic wrap to simulate the peritoneum draping over the uterus and bladder, creating a "bladder flap." The muscle layer is next (scored in the midline so it can be separated). An individual pyramidalis can be added, if one has enough fabric. The fascia material

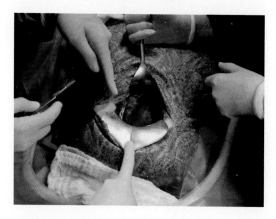

Fig. 9. Materials required for watermelon cesarean delivery model. (Courtesy of Lisa Harris, MD, and Dee Fenner, MD, Ann Arbor, MI.)
One large watermelon
One balloon filled with water (bladder)
Clear plastic wrap (peritoneum)
Thick red felt fabric (rectus and pyramidalis mm.)
Tough white fabric folded in half (two layers of fascia)
Quilting fluff (subcutaneous fat)
Quilted fabric (skin)
Rolled cardboard (symphysis)
Clear packing tape
Cesarean section drapes and instruments

is next, and then the skin. All of the fabric pieces are taped to the top and bottom of the watermelon.

Future trends in models

Although inexpensive models made from common materials will always have a place in medical education, the future for models looks bright. Animate models, such as the TraumaMan and the Human Patient Simulator, are on the horizon, with and without built-in interactive computer modules. Advances in robotic surgery (ie, DaVinci Surgical System, Intuitive Surgical, Sunnyvale, California) make it possible to combine a remote surgical model with a virtual reality model. This system uses binocular cameras to recreate the three-dimensional effect seen in open cases and puts them on a "heads-up" screen. This technology steepens the learning curve and allows a more junior trainee to perform at a higher level, especially with operative tasks.

Improvements in virtual reality technology will make realistic models that closely approximate operating on a human patient. First used commercially in flight simulators, this technology has been used for decades. To date, programs exist for cholecystectomy, laparoscopy, hysteroscopy, and neurosurgery.

References

[1] Austin F, Jones B. William Clift: the surgeon's apprentice. Ann R Coll Surg Engl 1978;60: 261–5.

[2] Rutkow IM. John Wyeth (1845–1922) and the postgraduate education and training of America's surgeons. Arch Surg 2002;137:748–9.

[3] Smith JJ, Gay SB, Maurer EJ, et al. Effect of Health Care Financing Administration regulations on radiology fellowship training. Acad Radiol 1999;6:126–31.

[4] McElearney ST, Saalwachter AR, Hedrick TL, et al. Effect of the 80-hour work week on cases performed by general surgery residents. Am Surg 2005;71:552–5.

[5] Wilson M, Palmer D. Facility construction. Animal Lab News 2005;4:20–3.

[6] Zikria BA. Exercise and drill boards for surgical training:10-year experience with a knot-tying board. Am J Surg 1981;141:612–3.

[7] Tritle NM, Haller JR, Gray SD. Aesthetic comparison of wound closure techniques in a porcine model. Laryngoscope 2001;111:1949–51.

[8] Gawande A. Education of a knife. In: Complications: a surgeon's notes on an imperfect science. New York: Henry Holt. p. 11–34.

[9] Bendavid R. The Shouldice technique: a canon in hernia repair. Can J Surg 1997;40: 199–205, 207.

[10] Maxwell JP, Masters RS, Eves FF. The role of working memory in motor learning and performance. Conscious Cogn 2003;12:376–402.

[11] Fenner DE. Training of a gynecologic surgeon. Obstet Gynecol 2005;105:193–6.

[12] Block EFJ, Lottenberg L, Flint L, et al. Use of human patient simulator for the Advanced Trauma Life Support Course. Am Surg 2002;68:648–51.

[13] Reznick RK. Teaching and testing technical skills. Am J Surg 1993;165:358–61.

[14] Viren NN, Matsumoto ED, Houston PL, et al. Fiberoptic orotracheal intubation on anesthetized patients: do manipulation skills learned on a simple model transfer into the operating room? Anesthesiol 2001;95:343–8.

[15] Reznick R, Regehr G, MacRae H, et al. Testing technical skill via an innovative bench station examination. Am J Surg 1997;180:226–30.

[16] Martin JA, Regehr G, Reznick R, et al. Objective structured assessment of technical skill (OSATS) for surgical residents. Br J Surg 1997;84:273–8.

[17] Goff BA, Nielsen PE, Lentz GM, et al. Surgical skills assessment: a blinded examination of obstetrics and gynecology residents. Am J Obstet Gynecol 2002;186:613–7.

[18] Van Rij AM, McDonald JR, Pettigrew RA, et al. Cusum as an aid to early assessment of the surgical trainee. Br J Surg 1995;82:1500–3.

[19] Myers DL, Arya LA, Verma A, et al. Pelvic anatomy for obstetrics and gynecology residents: an experimental study using clay models. Obstet Gynecol 2001;97:321–4.

[20] Cain JJ, Shirar E. A new method for teaching repair of perineal trauma at birth. Fam Med 1996;28:107–10.

[21] Gobbo RW, Canavan T. How to teach the perineal repair workshop in ALSO. In: Advanced life support in obstetrics instructor course syllabus. 3rd edition. Leawood (KS): American Academy of Family Physicians; 2002. p. 147–56.

ELSEVIER
SAUNDERS

Obstet Gynecol Clin N Am
33 (2006) 283–296

OBSTETRICS AND
GYNECOLOGY
CLINICS
OF NORTH AMERICA

Simulators and Virtual Reality in Surgical Education

Betty Chou, MD*, Victoria L. Handa, MD

*Department of Gynecology and Obstetrics, Johns Hopkins University School of Medicine,
Johns Hopkins Bayview Medical Center, Room 121 A1C, 4940 Eastern Avenue,
Baltimore, MD 21224, USA*

During residency training, surgical skills are taught and assessed using many different modalities, ranging from didactics, observation, simulators, and intraoperative education. Traditionally, surgical technical skills have been taught using the Halstedian apprenticeship model, centered on preceptor-based intraoperative instruction. The conventional paradigm of the apprenticeship model is no longer adequate for sustaining the gynecologist's training, maintenance, and assessment of these surgical skills. One reason for this change is the enormous increase in the number of highly technical procedures and minimally invasive surgeries introduced in recent years. Also, the resident work-hour limitations, increased interventional radiology procedures, medicinal advances, and super-subspecialization have reduced the number of operating room learning experiences for residents. In addition to medicolegal ramifications and risk to patients, training residents in the operating room is an enormous financial burden. The annual expense of educating and training surgical residents in the operating room was estimated to cost the medical system $53 million in 1997 [1]. Furthermore, the operating room may not be an ideal environment to learn surgical skills. The trainee may be tired, unprepared, or stressed, whereas the mentor may be unengaged or uninterested in teaching. The arena is inconsistent and incapable of being standardized. The apprenticeship model of surgical training is unstructured,

* Corresponding author.
E-mail address: bchou1@jhmi.edu (B. Chou).

0889-8545/06/$ – see front matter © 2006 Elsevier Inc. All rights reserved.
doi:10.1016/j.ogc.2006.01.007
obgyn.theclinics.com

unpredictable, and has been referred to as "education by random opportunity" [2]. Often, technical skills need repetition for mastery, which may not be practical or safe during actual surgeries [3]. For these many reasons, obstetrics and gynecology residency programs are adding surgical simulators to their surgical training curriculum.

Laparoscopic and hysteroscopic procedures add additional challenges to surgical training. Laparoscopy, in particular, requires complex hand-eye coordination, ambidexterity, understanding of the fulcrum effect, and depth perception [4]. These abilities can be challenging to master and often require extensive practice to become proficient. The paradigm of "see one, do one, teach one" cannot be safely applied to these technically advanced skills. It has been shown that inexperienced surgeons have significantly higher rates of operative complications when performing laparoscopic procedures [5]. It is critical to ensure that gynecologists have adequate instruction. Current inadequacies in surgical skills instruction is evident when only 18% of surveyed surgical residents believe their training program has adequately prepared them to perform advanced laparoscopic procedures [6]. Furthermore, there is a need for additional and novel training opportunities for postgraduate surgical training, because new techniques will be developed after an obstetrician-gynecologist has completed his or her residency training. Surgeons already out in practice need a format to receive instruction and undergo assessments on these new advanced skills.

Simulators allow a surgeon safely to overcome the learning curve of a new technique before practicing on a living patient. For example, a variety of surgical procedures can be practiced on a human cadaver, thereby simulating real surgery. Cadaver models have accurate anatomy and realism, but are expensive, scarce, and have altered tissue compliance. Live animal models have comparable anatomy and well-established use with surgical training, but the challenges of establishing an animal training laboratory include substantial overhead, the technical complexity of animal care, and important ethical considerations. Additionally, animal and cadaver models are not practical options for repetitive tasks or practice. Mechanical simulators, also called box trainers or conventional trainers, have long been used to teach laparoscopic skills. Box trainers are a popular alternative to animal and cadaver models, because they are less expensive and more convenient. Computer-based virtual reality simulators are relatively new to surgical education but are growing in popularity. Virtual reality simulators allow more independent instruction and objective immediate feedback for more reliable, unbiased assessment of psychomotor skills. These qualities have been shown to enhance surgical skills instruction in highly technical skills. Virtual reality simulators allow risk-free training in a nonthreatening environment where trainees can repetitively practice a surgical skill without squandering expensive resources [2]. This article presents the relative pros and cons of virtual reality trainers for training novice gynecologists, for assessing surgical competence, and for allowing experienced surgeons to develop new surgical techniques.

Goals of simulators

In surgical education, box trainers and virtual reality trainers have been used to train specific psychomotor skills and to assess performance. Achieving these objectives depends on three essential principles: (1) validity, (2) reliability, and (3) feasibility [7].

Validity refers to whether the assessment modality measures what it intends to measure. Predictive validity refers to how well the assessment test predicts future performance. Construct validity refers to how well the test is measuring the specific trait in question. Often the most important feature, face validity, refers to how well the examination reflects what happens in the real world [8]. Validity depends on realistic tasks that are technically similar to real conditions.

Reliability refers to the precision of the assessment tool and the reproducibility of the results. It allows objective assessment of performance. Finally, feasibility refers to its practicality. Feasibility improves when the simulator demands little time, money, or effort. The most feasible modalities are easy to perform, require little guidance from instructors, use inexpensive equipment and materials, allow independent practice, and do not require much time [8].

Box trainers

Many training programs use box trainers to enhance the surgical curriculum, either for practicing or assessing laparoscopic skills. Most box trainer simulators use actual laparoscopic equipment, including laparoscope, camera, light source, trocars, and laparoscopic instruments, placed through an opaque cover over the training area. Predetermined tasks are developed to mimic a specific psychomotor skill or actual surgical procedure. Ideally, the trainee performs the laparoscopic tasks under direct guidance of an experienced mentor for instruction and feedback. The length of time required to complete the task is recorded and the number of errors (definition of errors are also predetermined) is reflected as a penalty.

This general simulator format has been used by many obstetric-gynecology and surgery residency programs. There has been much interest in trying to verify that training on a box trainer does indeed improve laparoscopic skills and that this improvement can be translated to the operating room. Although little data can be found on this subject in the obstetric-gynecology literature, extensive research in this area can be found in the general surgery literature.

Considerable research has been devoted to studying the McGill Inanimate System for Training and Evaluation of Laparoscopic Skills program (MISTELS). The program is composed of a series of seven laparoscopic tasks: (1) pegboard patterns (transferring); (2) pattern cutting; (3) clip application; (4) ligating loop; (5) mesh placement; (6) intracorporeal knot; and (7) extracorporeal knot [4,9]. Derossis and coworkers [4] demonstrated that performance scores on the MISTELS tasks were significantly correlated with level of training or expertise, supporting the construct validity of the simulator.

Research suggests that supervised practice with box trainers improves surgical performance. In the earliest research [4,10,11], practice and repetition with the simulator led to improved performance as measured by a structured set of tasks performed with the box trainer. It is not surprising, however, that practicing with the box trainer leads to improvement in performing tasks with that simulator. The next question is whether those skills can transfer out of the simulator environment. Using an animal model to assess intracorporeal knot tying, Rosser and colleagues [11] found significant improvement in the time required to complete the intracorporeal knot after practicing three coordination drills with a box trainer (rope pass, cup drop, triangle transfer). In a similar study, Fried and coworkers [9] demonstrated that there were significant improvements in nearly all in vivo tasks in the group that received box training when compared with the group with no training. These studies suggest that box trainer simulators do improve laparoscopic skills.

The ultimate question to be answered is whether this type of training improves performance in the operating room with real patients. Scott and coworkers [12] randomized surgical residents to a box trainer group or to a no training group. All residents in both groups received routine surgical instruction as part of typical residency training. Using a global assessment tool for laparoscopic cholecystectomy on an actual patient, investigators found that the training group demonstrated significantly greater improvement in overall global assessment scores when compared with the group with no training. The areas of improvement were respect for tissue, instrument handling, use of assistants, and overall performance. No improvement was seen in four other criteria: (1) flow of operation, (2) knowledge of instruments, (3) knowledge of procedure, and (4) time and motion. Box trainers are more useful in improving specific technical skills than in improving the overall conduct of the surgical procedure.

Virtual reality surgical simulators

Supported by the success of flight simulation for the training of pilots, virtual reality training in surgical skills is growing in interest and popularity. Virtual reality simulators are computer-based, consisting of a frame holding two standard laparoscopic instruments and a digital foot pedal all electronically linked to a personal computer. The software constructs a virtual environment seen on the computer screen, which shows position and movement of the laparoscopic instruments in real time. As the participant performs a task, the computer records every movement and error for analysis [13]. The learner is provided with feedback regarding various aspects of performance. The programs vary considerably from low-fidelity simple object-oriented task simulation (Fig. 1) to high-resolution three-dimensional graphics, which constructs a virtual anatomically accurate

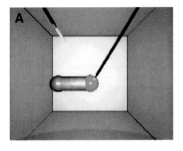 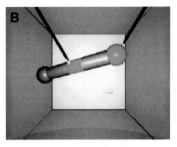

Fig. 1. The StretchClip task in a virtual reality surgical simulator (MIST 2). (*A*) Grasp tube. (*B*) Stretch tube to desired length and apply clip. (*From* Gor M, McCloy R, Stone R, et al. Virtual reality laparoscopic simulator for assessment in gynaecology. BJOG 2003;110(2):181–7.)

setting compiled from actual CT or MRI scans (Fig. 2) [14]. The most advanced systems provide haptic or tactile feedback.

Much of the virtual reality training research has used the minimally invasive surgical trainer–virtual reality (MIST-VR) system. This simple object skill-oriented simulator is comprised of six tasks without haptic feedback: (1) acquire and place (grasp virtual sphere and place in virtual box); (2) transfer and place (grasp sphere, transfer, and place in box); (3) traversal (grasp alternately the segments of a virtual pipe); (4) withdraw and insert (grasp sphere, touch, withdraw instrument, and repeat); (5) diathermy (apply diathermy to targets on sphere); and (6) manipulation and diathermy (combines the fourth and fifth task) [13,15].

As with the box trainer, the key questions include whether practice with the virtual reality trainer helps the learner acquire basic technical skills and whether this improves performance in the operating room. In research studies, practice with a virtual reality trainer consistently improved basic skills, such as manipulating objects. Gallagher and coworkers [16] and Grantcharov and coworkers [17] both demonstrated that previous laparoscopic experience was highly correlated with performance on the MIST-VR simulator, substantiating its construct validity. Gallagher and coworkers [18] demonstrated that MIST-VR training improved the ability of endoscopic novices to perform a box trainer cutting task. These novices were more likely to use both hands effectively if randomized to the group receiving MIST-VR training beforehand. This suggests that virtual reality training can improve laparoscopic skills (at least in a training laboratory).

Most importantly, can virtual reality training improve operating room performance? Recent randomized, blinded, control trials have addressed this issue. Grantcharov and colleagues [15] assessed surgical residents during a laparoscopic cholecystectomy (on an actual patient) using a global assessment scale. Residents received conventional residency training and were randomly assigned to additional MIST-VR training or no simulator training. Those with virtual reality training had significantly shorter operating times, fewer errors, and better

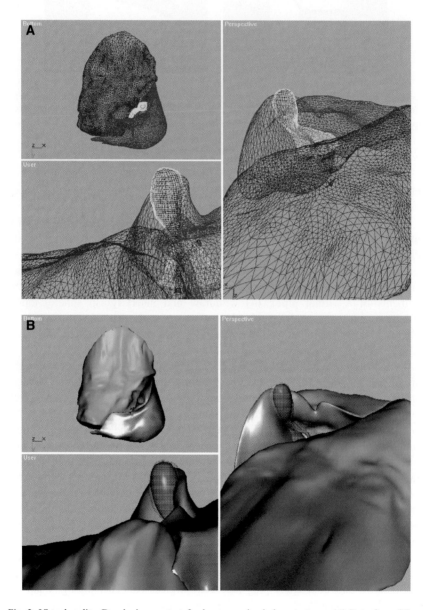

Fig. 2. Virtual reality. Developing content for laparoscopic cholecystectomy. (*A*) Data from CT are used to create a polygonal mesh, simulating gallbladder anatomy. (*B*) With contour applied. (*C*) With texture applied. (*D*) Finished simulated environment. (Reproduced from Simbionix LAP Mentor with permission of Simbionix Corporation, Cleveland, Ohio.)

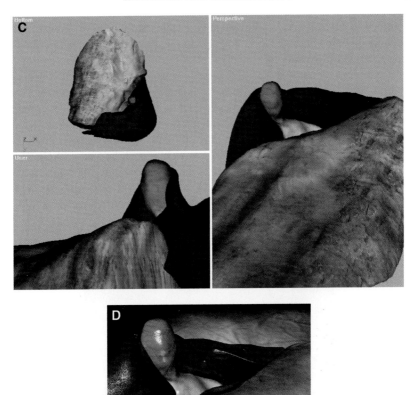

Fig. 2 (*continued*).

economy of motion when compared with those with no training. Similarly, other studies also showed that residents randomized to receive MIST-VR training also performed better at laparoscopic cholecystectomy [5,19]. Ahlberg and co-workers [20], however, were not able to verify this association with MIST-VR training of medical students. Medical students trained on MIST-VR did not demonstrate improved operative skills on an animal model when compared with those with no virtual reality training. These conflicting findings weaken the conviction that virtual reality simulators have proved use. Admittedly, it is difficult to compare these studies because all have inconsistent training regimens and evaluation methods.

Although nearly all of the virtual reality simulator data is found in the general surgery literature, a handful of articles devoted to virtual reality training applicable to gynecology have appeared. Gynecologic surgery is not simply general surgery performed in the pelvis; new virtual reality systems are needed to simulate pelvic anatomy and unique tasks specific to gynecology. Researchers have described the used of virtual reality training systems for laparoscopic bilateral tubal ligation and hysteroscopic interventions [21,22]. Other virtual reality training products for obstetrics and gynecology have been newly released or are in the development phase, including hysteroscopic resection of a myoma (Fig. 3), endometrial ablation, and laparoscopic removal of a tubal ectopic pregnancy. Furthermore, some virtual reality simulator models may allow for skills to be transferred to an obstetrics and gynecology specific task. For example, skills learned from virtual reality training in epidural injections or peritoneal lavage may be transferable to the performance of an amniocentesis [23]. As more interest arises for virtual reality training in obstetrics and gynecology, more virtual reality simulator programs will be developed.

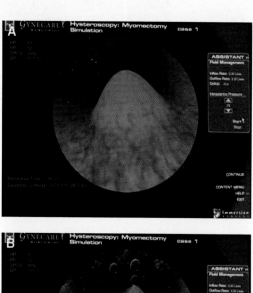

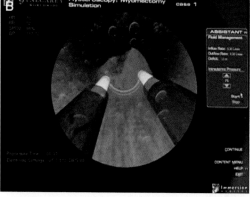

Fig. 3. Virtual reality simulation of hysteroscopic resection of a myoma. (*A*) Submucosal myoma seen hysteroscopically. (*B*) Hysteroscopic resection of myoma. (Courtesy of Immersion Corporation, San Jose, California, © 2005 Immersion Corporation, all rights reserved.)

Virtual reality trainers versus box trainers

Although most are convinced that simulators are useful training tools for highly technical surgical skills, there is not much consensus on which simulator modality is most effective. Many training programs do not have the resources to equip their curriculum with both box trainers and virtual reality trainers. The logical question arises: which simulator is better?

Numerous investigations [13,24,25] compared the technical skills of trainees after being randomized to a no training group, a box trainer group, or a virtual reality trainer group. The effects of the training randomization were assessed by the graded performance on a standardized box trainer task. Consistently, both training groups did significantly better at the box trainer task when compared with the group with no simulator training. No significant differences were seen, however, between the box trainer group and the virtual reality trainer group. Both improved skills equally well above those with no training, suggesting that there is no advantage of one type of simulator trainer over the other. Although these studies imply that these two modalities of training are equivalent with respect to the performance of basic tasks in a surgical laboratory, one cannot assume these finding are necessarily echoed in an actual operating room, which is the most important query.

Hamilton and coworkers [26] tackled this exact question in his research trial. He randomized 50 surgery residents to box training or virtual reality training. After the designated training, participants had their technical skills assessed during an actual laparoscopic cholecystectomy. The virtual reality training significantly improved resident performance during operating room case, whereas training with a box trainer did not improve performance. The authors concluded that virtual reality training is superior. In a 2005 study [27], surgeon performance was compared after practice with either a box trainer or a high-fidelity virtual reality simulator. In that study, performance was assessed in an animal model. Again, investigators found that the virtual reality trainer was superior. They speculated that the simple box trainer tasks did not demonstrate enough realism for complex tasks. It allowed only minimal multidirectional movement and did not respond to extreme force on the inanimate objects. In contrast, the high-fidelity virtual reality system had simulated tissue that had multidirectional, dynamic motion that ruptured if handled with excessive tension. They concluded that the low-fidelity box trainer was adequate for basic tasks, but virtual reality was superior for learning more complicated, two-handed, coordinated skills. The question that remains is whether the additional benefit of virtual reality is worth the additional cost above the traditional box trainer [27].

Cost considerations

The main argument against virtual reality trainers is the high cost associated with such systems. The expense of a virtual reality simulator is directly proportional with its level of sophistication. Satava [14] describes the five components fundamental to virtual reality: (1) fidelity (does it seem real); (2) object properties (organs deform with pressure or fall with gravity); (3) interactivity (instruments interact with organs realistically); (4) sensory input (is there force feedback); and (5) reactivity (organs must react appropriately, such as bleeding or leaking). Improvements to these properties are associated with significantly higher costs to the training system and can be prohibitive to its widespread use.

Although the box trainer is less expensive to set up, it does have some hidden expenses. Unlike the virtual reality simulator, the box trainer has tasks that usually consume materials that need to be bought and replaced. More importantly, it requires more manpower. The tasks usually require at least two participants: one to perform the assigned task and a mentor (who gives instruction and feedback). The feedback component is critical to learning and perfecting surgical skills but is absent without the presence of a skilled surgeon mentor. The additional personnel add costs to the department, both in time and money. Because feedback and assessment are typically an intrinsic function of virtual reality simulators, learners can benefit from unsupervised practice with a virtual reality simulator. It can be difficult to compare the long-term costs of virtual reality with conventional box trainers. To date, there has been no detailed cost analysis of the use of these types of simulators in gynecology training. To appreciate fully the cost-effectiveness of either simulator, the transfer efficiency ratio must be determined. Flight simulation data have revealed that 1 hour of simulation training equals half an hour of in-flight training (transfer efficiency ratio=2:1); however, the transfer efficiency ratio for simulation training of surgical skills has not been established [24,25].

Which simulator do surgical trainees prefer?

Regardless of any proved efficacy or cost-effectiveness, trainees seem to prefer the box trainers. Through questionnaires, surgery residents indicate that they favor box trainers over virtual reality trainers because it is "more realistic," citing more tactile feedback and better depth perception [26]. This is despite greater improvement in surgeon performance with the virtual reality training in this particular study. Because of its relative affordability, most of the virtual reality simulators used for training today are systems that have low-fidelity tasks that lack haptic feedback. These perceived shortcomings have affected the eagerness of trainees to use the virtual reality simulators. Other research has confirmed this attitude. Madan and coworkers [28] demonstrated that trainees believe that box trainers help more, are more interesting, and should be chosen over virtual reality trainers if only one trainer is permitted. They also believe that the box trainers were more realistic, because they use real laparoscopic equipment. These opinions may affect trainee use of these simulator modules. Will residents be motivated to use the virtual reality above the box trainer if they do not like it more? These many issues are clouding the answer as to which simulator modality is best for each training program.

Assessing surgical skills and feedback

Perhaps the most promising role for virtual reality simulator is in the assessment of surgical competency. Currently, most gynecology faculty evaluate their residents using recall-based, end-of-rotation assessments that has been shown to have poor reliability and validity [29]. Also, valid assessment tools for physician credentialing and recertification are lacking. For example, surgical privileges are often based on the reported number of times a surgeon has previously performed a specific procedure, rather than the surgeon's competence. Simulators offer the promise of a more objective and reliable method to evaluate surgeon competency and skill.

Both box trainers and virtual reality trainers can be used in the assessment of surgical competence [4,10,16,30]. These two types of simulators, however, offer very different types of assessment and feedback. With a box trainer, a mentor or instructor must be present to assess the surgeon's performance and to provide feedback. Surgical trainees may be asked to complete a series of structured tasks, such as MISTELS. To minimize the bias introduced by the relationship between the evaluator and the student, the simulation can be recorded and viewed later. The resulting assessment, however, is typically a subjective assessment. This method of evaluation and feedback can be fraught with bias and poor reliability.

In contrast, the virtual reality simulator is an objective assessment tool. Data from the performance can be analyzed by the computer to evaluate for accuracy and errors, completion time, efficacy of using the right or left hand, and economy of motion and diathermy [31]. This unbiased feedback is innate to the system and is not dependant on an outside observer or evaluator. By providing immediate feedback, virtual reality systems can aid the learner in self-assessment and can guide further practice. The assessment and feedback features of virtual reality simulator systems make it a valuable component of surgical training. For example, Grantcharov and coworkers [32] evaluated surgery residents assessed on six MIST-VR tasks. The following day these same residents were evaluated on total errors and economy of motion during a laparoscopic cholecystectomy in an animal model. Performance during the laparoscopic surgery was strongly correlated with performance on the virtual reality tasks. Similarly, Ahlberg and coworkers [20] showed that those medical students who performed well on the MIST-VR also did well on an animal model. Additionally, this simulator can detect a decline in surgeon performance caused by the effects of sleep deprivation or alcohol intoxication. Under such conditions, intoxicated or sleep-deprived surgeons consistently make more errors than unimpaired surgeons [33,34]. Virtual reality seems to be an objective and reliable assessment modality for laparoscopic skills.

Most of the research regarding the assessment abilities of virtual reality has been located in the general surgery field; however, there have also been some literature exploring the use of virtual reality in assessing surgical skills in gynecology. Gor and colleagues [35] studied the use of MIST 2 (a second-generation virtual reality laparoscopic training simulator). MIST 2 is similar to MIST-VR, but has two additional tasks that are more geared toward gynecologic procedures. The StretchClip task is analogous to a laparoscopic sterilization technique (see Fig. 1). The StretchDiathermy task is analogous to a laparoscopic removal of an ectopic pregnancy. Using MIST-2, Gor and colleagues [35] found that the MIST 2 is an objective assessment tool for evaluating laparoscopic skills in gynecologists.

Future directions

Virtual reality simulators evaluate psychomotor skills during a standardized task, allowing trainees to be assessed and compared objectively. This assessment tool may be able to identify potential residency candidates who may not perform well in the operating room. As many as 10% of medical students may not have the innate abilities to acquire satisfactory surgical skills [35]. Gallagher and coworkers [16] showed that a small subset of medical students had significantly poorer performance scores on MIST-VR tasks and that this group was unable to demonstrate any pattern of improvement despite practice when compared with the other better performing medical students. For those who cannot demonstrate proficiency, a simulator test may help guide career choices.

Additionally, virtual reality simulator testing may be used as a tool for certification or recertification throughout a surgeon's career. As more and more surgical techniques are introduced into gynecology, there is a growing need to ensure surgical competence, even in the experienced surgeon. Too often a surgeon is permitted to perform a new skill on a patient simply because they have practiced the procedure a specified number of times, not because proficiency has been proved. Simulator testing may be an objective method for determining that a surgeon has the adequate skills to perform a procedure safely. Passing a simulator test may be required before advancing to the next stage of training or getting privileges to perform a highly technical procedure. For example, research is being conducted to explore the clinical outcomes if surgeons are permitted to place a carotid stent in a patient only after establishing a level of proficiency on the virtual reality trainer [36]. Clinical outcomes will be compared between patients who received a stent from an experienced physician and those who received their stent from a virtual reality trained (but less experienced) physician. This type of posttraining competency testing also may be applied to new or complicated gynecologic procedures.

Summary

The apprenticeship model for learning complex surgical skills is no longer adequate. Simulators must be added to the obstetrics and gynecology training curriculum to familiarize a surgeon to an advanced technique safely. Virtual reality trainers are a relatively new type of training simulator, but have shown tremendous promise for superior training of highly complex surgical skills, objective assessment of ability, and application as a tool for certification. The virtual reality systems are considerably more expensive than traditional box trainers, however, and their use outside of the general surgery discipline has only been modestly explored. More research is needed to investigate and support the use of virtual reality trainers in the field of obstetrics and gynecology.

References

[1] Bridges M, Diamond D. The financial impact of teaching surgical residents in the operating room. Am J Surg 1999;177:28–32.

[2] Cosman P, Cregan P, Martin C, et al. Virtual reality simulators: current status in acquisition and assessment of surgical skills. Aust N Z J Surg 2002;72:30–4.

[3] Haluck R, Krummel T. Computers and virtual reality for surgical education in the 21st century. Arch Surg 2000;135:786–92.

[4] Derossis A, Fried G, Abrahamowicz M, et al. Development of a model for training and evaluation of laparoscopic skills. Am J Surg 1998;175:482–7.

[5] Seymour N, Gallagher A, Roman S, et al. Virtual reality training improves operating room performance- results of a randomized, double-blinded study. Ann Surg 2002;236:458–64.

[6] Chiasson P, Pace D, Schlacta C, et al. Minimally invasive surgery training in Canada: a survey of general surgery residents. Surg Endosc 2003;17:371–7.

[7] Reznick R. Teaching and testing technical skills. Am J Surg 1993;165:358–61.

[8] Grantcharov T, Bardram L, Funch-Jensen P, et al. Assessment of technical surgical skills. Eur J Surg 2002;168:139–44.

[9] Fried G, Derossis A, Bothwell J, et al. Comparison of laparoscopic performance in vivo with performance measured in a laparoscopic simulator. Surg Endosc 1999;13:1077–81.

[10] Derossis A, Bothwell J, Sigman H, et al. The effect of practice on performance in a laparoscopic simulator. Surg Endosc 1998;12:1117–20.

[11] Rosser J, Rosser L, Savalgi R. Skill acquisition and assessment for laparoscopic surgery. Arch Surg 1997;132:200–4.

[12] Scott D, Bergen P, Rege R, et al. Laparoscopic training on bench models: better and more cost effective than operating room experience? J Am Coll Surg 2000;191:272–83.

[13] Kothari S, Kaplan B, DeMaria E, et al. Training in laparoscopic suturing skills using a new computer-based virtual reality simulator (MIST-VR) provides results comparable to those with an established pelvic trainer system. J Laparoendosc Adv Surg Tech A 2002;12:167–73.

[14] Satava R. Virtual reality surgical simulator. Surg Endosc 1993;7:203–5.

[15] Grantcharov T, Kristiansen V, Bendix J, et al. Randomized clinical trail of virtual reality simulation for laparoscopic skills training. Br J Surg 2004;91:146–50.

[16] Gallagher A, Lederman A, McGlade K, et al. Discriminative validity of the minimally invasive surgical trainer in virtual reality (MIST-VR) using criteria levels based on expert performance. Surg Endosc 2004;18:660–5.

[17] Grantcharov T, Bardram L, Funch-Jensen P, et al. Learning curves and the impact of previous

operative experience on performance on a virtual reality simulator to test laparoscopic surgical skills. Am J Surg 2003;285:146–9.

[18] Gallagher A, McClure N, McGuigan J, et al. Virtual reality training in laparoscopic surgery: a preliminary assessment of minimally invasive surgical trainer virtual reality (MIST VR). Endoscopy 1999;31:310–3.

[19] Schijven M, Jakimowicz J, Broeders M, et al. The Eindhoven laparoscopic cholecystectomy training course. Improving operating room performance using virtual reality training: results from the first EAES accredited virtual reality training curriculum. Surg Endosc 2005;19(9):1220–6.

[20] Ahlberg G, Heikkinen T, Iselius L, et al. Does training in a virtual reality simulator improve surgical performance? Surg Endosc 2002;16:126–9.

[21] Sung W, Fung C, Chen A, et al. The assessment of stability and reliability of a virtual reality-based laparoscopic gynecology simulation system. Eur J Gynaecol Oncol 2003;24:143–6.

[22] Muller-Wittig W, Bisler A, Bockholt U, et al. LAHYSTOTRAIN development and evaluation of a complex training system for hysteroscopy. Stud Health Technol Inform 2001;81:336–40.

[23] Letterie G. How virtual reality may enhance training in obstetrics and gynecology. Am J Obstet Gynecol 2002;187:S37–40.

[24] Torkington J, Smith G, Rees B, et al. Skill transfer from virtual reality to a real laparoscopic task. Surg Endosc 2001;15:1076–9.

[25] Munz Y, Kumar B, Moorthy K, et al. Laparoscopic virtual reality and box trainers: is one superior to the other? Surg Endosc 2004;18:485–94.

[26] Hamilton E, Scott D, Fleming J, et al. Comparison of video trainer and virtual reality training systems on acquisition of laparoscopic skills. Surg Endosc 2002;16:406–11.

[27] Youngblood P, Srivastava S, Curet M, et al. Comparison of training on two laparoscopic simulators and assessment of skill transfer to surgical performance. J Am Coll Surg 2005;200: 546–51.

[28] Madan A, Frantzides C, Tebbitt C, et al. Participants' opinions of laparoscopic training devices after a basic laparoscopic training course. Am J Surg 2005;189:758–61.

[29] Mandel L, Lentz G, Goff B. Teaching and evaluating surgical skills. Obstet Gynecol 2000;95:783–5.

[30] Derossis A, Antoniuk M, Fried G. Evaluation of laparoscopic skills: a 2 year follow-up during residency training. Can J Surg 1999;42:293–6.

[31] McCloy R, Stone R. Science, medicine, and the future: virtual reality in surgery. BMJ 2001; 323:912–5.

[32] Grantcharov T, Rosenberg J, Pahle E, et al. Virtual reality computer simulation: an objective method for the evaluation of laparoscopic surgical skills. Surg Endosc 2001;15:242–4.

[33] Taffinder N, McManus I, Gul Y, et al. Effect of sleep deprivation of surgeons' dexterity on laparoscopy simulator. Lancet 1998;352:1191.

[34] Brunner W, Korndorffer J, Sierra R, et al. Laparoscopic virtual reality training: are 30 repetitions enough? J Surg Res 2004;122:150–6.

[35] Gor M, McCloy R, Stone R, et al. Virtual reality laparoscopic simulator for assessment in gynaecology. BJOG 2003;110:181–7.

[36] Gallagher A, Cates C. Approval of virtual reality training for carotid stenting: what this means for procedural-based medicine. JAMA 2004;292:3024–6.

ELSEVIER
SAUNDERS

Obstet Gynecol Clin N Am
33 (2006) 297–304

OBSTETRICS AND
GYNECOLOGY
CLINICS
OF NORTH AMERICA

Mental Practice and Acquisition of Motor Skills: Examples from Sports Training and Surgical Education

Rebecca G. Rogers, MD

Department of Obstetrics and Gynecology, University of New Mexico Health Sciences Center,
MSC10 5580, ACC Fourth Floor, Albuquerque, NM 87131–0001, USA

Mental preparation is important for the performance of both physical and mental tasks, and its efficacy is well documented in the sports literature. In its purest form, mental practice is the cognitive rehearsal of a task without overt physical movement [1], although some researchers have added physical movements to enhance the effects of the mental practice [2]. Mental practice has been variously termed "imaginary practice," "covert rehearsal," "conceptualization," or "mental imagery rehearsal" [1,3]. It can be used to enhance the acquisition of new technical skills, and increase emotional preparedness to perform in stressful situations, both qualities applicable to the training of surgical residents.

Most surgeons report going over procedures in "their mind's eye" [3] in preparation for the operating room, but surprisingly little research has examined the effect of these interventions on surgical trainees' operating room performance. This article reviews the theories of how mental practice impacts acquisition of technical skills and the literature of the use of mental practice in sports training. The application of mental practice to surgical skills training with particular emphasis on the use of mental practice as part of the surgical training curriculum at the University of New Mexico Health Sciences' Department of Obstetrics and Gynecology is also delineated.

E-mail address: rrogers@salud.unm.edu

doi:10.1016/j.ogc.2006.02.004

obgyn.theclinics.com

Mental representations: a dual coding approach

Representation is defined as a likeness, portrait, image, or description, and can be either physical or mental. Representations are symbolic and vary in abstractness [4]. One theory postulates that there are two classes of phenomena handled cognitively by different systems: one specialized for the representation and processing of information concerning nonverbal objects and events, and the other specializing with language. The nonverbal symbolic subsystem is the "imagery system" because its critical functions include the analysis of scenes and the generation mental images. The second system can be categorized as "verbal." Both play a critical role in representations.

Mental practice using the imagery system impacts both cognition and motivation [5]. How greatly it changes performance of motor skills or emotional responses to stressful situations varies with the individual because different images mean different things to different people [6] and may elicit different physiologic and emotional reactions [7].

Why does mental practice improve motor skills? Two theories are postulated. The psychoneuromuscular theory purports that mental practice strengthens muscle memory by having muscles fire in the correct sequence for a movement, without executing the movement itself [8]. The second theory is that mental practice imagery produces mental blueprints for movement patterns and that mental rehearsal of the blueprints allows movements to become familiar and automatic [8]. Acquisition of motor skills and their application to complex cognitive performance is not limited to only execution of actual movements but also requires that the motor skills be successfully executed in a stressful situation. Successful implementation of motor skills also involves goal setting. A sports model of mental practice imagery has been proposed that incorporates both cognitive, or skills acquisition, and motivational theories. This theory is reviewed in the following section.

Sports imagery theory

Five areas of imagery have been identified in the sports literature: (1) motivational specific, (2) motivational general–mastery, (3) motivational general–arousal, (4) cognitive specific, and (5) cognitive general (Table 1). Motivational specific imagery represents specific goal setting, such as imaging winning an event, or being congratulated for a successful performance. Motivational general–mastery imagery represents effective coping and mastery of challenging situations. Motivational general–arousal imagery represents the feelings that are needed to be effective (eg, feeling relaxed, aroused, or anxious). The two cognitive imagery areas of sports imagery are specific to motor skills; cognitive specific is used to imagine a specific skill, such a throwing a ball, whereas cognitive general may be thought of as the game plan that links together specific motor skills. Validation of the use of these imagery models has been proved with

Table 1
Model of imagery used in sports training

Type of imagery	Definition	Examples
Cognitive		
Cognitive specific	Learning a specific task	Throwing a ball
Cognitive general	Linking task together	Executing a complex play in football
Motivational		
Motivational specific	Specific goal setting	Winning an event
Motivational general - mastery	Coping in competition	Being mentally tough and confident
Motivational general - arousal	Feeling relaxed, stressed, arousal, and so forth	Relaxing when taking a foul shot during a basketball game

a scale that measured the use of these techniques by athletes. The model was shown to have good construct validity and internal consistency when tested [9].

Cognitive specific imagery or the imagery of skills has been proved to improve performance of skills over a wide variety of sports including both fine motor skills and gross motor tasks. Cognitive specific imagery improves performance of specific tasks better than other types of imagery; studies of beginning runners who imagined all the movements of running performed better than runners who imagined themselves crossing the finish line [10]. Another study of sit-up performance showed that participants who imagined performing the sit-ups did better than those that imagined themselves as feeling confident when performing sit-ups [11] (one wonders if the imagery could also improve abdominal wall strength). Cognitive general imagery that links specific motor skills into game plans has been shown to be effective for rehearsing football plays [12], gymnastic routines [13], and slalom races [14].

Motivational general strategies have been used to enhance an athletes' self-confidence by imagining overcoming difficult situations and feeling in control [7]. Motivational specific strategies may also affect motivation and effort. For example, beginning golfers who imagined a successful performance outcome (sinking a putt) set higher goals and practiced longer hours than those that imaged a specific motor skill [7]. Imagery has also been used in sports to "psych up" before an event or to relax in stressful situations. One study has shown that imagining "your heart rate increasing" or "butterflies in your stomach" did in fact increase heart rates [15].

Imagery techniques progress with the advancing skill of the athlete; novices tend to focus on cognitive specific skills, because they are learning specific movements. Cognitive general skills are used by more advanced athletes to link the skills together, whereas the motivational and arousal techniques are used to improve overall performance [14].

Mental practice does impact performance, but physical practice is better because actual physical repetition of a task results in faster mastery. When physical practice is impossible, expensive, or unethical, however, mental imagery may be useful. Examples of situations where mental practice is useful includes after injuries, when physical practice is impossible, or when expensive equipment may not be available for practice. Additionally, physical practice may be unethical because it places either the person practicing or other individuals at risk. Examples of the latter include airline pilots and novice surgeons where physical practice on live subjects places the subjects at risk.

For mental imagery to be effective, the learner must be familiar with the task before the imagery session [1]. It is not useful to subjects mentally to practice a complex dance move, if the individual does not dance or has not seen similar movements; therefore, some direct observation of a task aids the individual in mental practice. A meta-analysis of mental imagery has also shown that mental practice improves tasks with a large cognitive component better than tasks that are purely physical. For example, such tasks as constructing cardboard boxes that are simply repetitive but do not require cognitive input are less likely to improve with mental practice than such tasks as running a football game plan that require larger cognitive input.

Mental practice is best when the actual performance immediately follows the imagery session; however, some improvement in the performance of tasks has been documented up to 21 days after mental imagery sessions [1]. The effect of mental imagery on motor skill acquisition is inversely proportional to the length of the imagery session; an analysis of sports literature suggests that effect is negligible in sessions more than 20 minutes in length [1]. Mental practice is best when it occurs immediately before physical practice and when it is brief and focused on the skills and emotive responses particular to the individual.

Use of mental practice imagery for improvement of motor skills is not limited to sports. It has also been shown to be effective in relearning motor skills after cerebral infarction. One example is a trial where 46 patients were randomized to receive 15 sessions of either mental imagery or conventional functional training to relearn daily tasks after cerebral infarction. Patients in the mental imagery–based group showed better relearning of tasks compared with the control group. They also demonstrated a greater ability to retain the skill 1 month after their mental imagery session and could better transfer relearned skills to other untrained tasks [16].

Predictors of surgical skills

Surgical skill combines both cognitive and motivational elements. Predictors of surgical skills are not necessarily the same predictors of what makes successful medical students. One study evaluated 120 general surgery residents with a neuropsychologic test battery and more traditional measures, such as the Medical College Admission Test and National Board scores. Residents were then rated on surgical skills by attending physicians during 1445 procedures. Surgical skill was most closely related to neuropsychologic factors including complex visuospatial organization, stress tolerance, psychomotor abilities. Surgical skills as assessed by attending physicians were not correlated to National Board scores and negatively correlated with Medical College Admission Test scores. The authors conclude that "... the ability to acquire knowledge, although necessary, is not a sufficient condition for operative skill" [17]. This may account for the approximately 10% of medical students who do not improve motor skills despite practice with a virtual reality simulator [18]. Because of the link between surgical skills and visuospatial organization, stress tolerance, and psychomotor skills, mental practice may be particularly suited to training surgical residents.

Mental imagery and surgical skills

The literature evaluating the use of mental imagery to teach surgical skills includes two recently published trials. The first is a study of teaching basic surgical skills to medical students. After a 1-hour lecture and demonstration of suturing on a pig's foot, 65 second-year medical students were randomized to three different groups. The first group had three sessions of physical practice suturing a pig's foot; the second group had two sessions of physical practice, and one session of mental practice imagery; and the third had one session of physical practice and two sessions of imagery rehearsal. The primary outcome measure was performance of surgery on a live rabbit after the training period. Although a power analysis was not performed because the study was performed on a convenience sample of students, no significant differences were noted between the three groups in skill acquisition. The authors conclude that mental imagery, combined with physical practice, may be economically beneficial in surgical skills training [3]. In addition to this study the authors also report on unpublished data of a trial with the same population of medical students that showed that guided imagery was superior to studying text in learning basic surgical skills [3].

A second study randomized 44 first-year medical students to mental imagery; mental imagery with kinesiology (the addition of movement to mental practice); or to standard Advanced Trauma Life Support training in learning emergency cricothyrotomy on a mannequin. The students underwent a 1-hour training session and 1 week later were tested with an Objective Structured Clinical Examination. The authors conclude that mental imagery with kinesiology improved results when compared with standard Advanced Trauma Life Support training [2]. Both of these studies illustrate that mental imagery may be equivalent to physical practice and offers cheaper and ethically sound ways for novice surgeons to prepare before operating on live patients.

Does mental imagery for teaching surgical skills make sense?

Mental imagery for teaching surgical skills has been used unofficially for years for the teaching of surgical skills. Many surgeons report that they mentally review cases before a surgery on a routine basis. The review may be on the cognitive general level with linking specific steps of a procedure, or more cognitive specific, such as placing a difficult suture or performing a difficult dissection. Learning surgical skills involves many gross and fine motor skills that are cognitively demanding. Mental practice imagery can be used not only to help with the acquisition of motor skills that are important to the performance of surgery, but also with stress management that can hinder trainees' ability to learn in live surgery.

The University of New Mexico's experience

For the past 5 years, the urogynecology division at the University of New Mexico has included mental practice imagery in the preoperative preparation of cases. The imagery sessions are typically performed the day before the surgery and per resident last approximately 20 minutes in length. The imagery sessions are tailored to the expertise of the resident or fellow; second-year residents are required to explain how they would place a suture or hold a clamp, whereas more senior residents and fellows are linking specific motor tasks to performance of complex surgical reconstructions. Before the imagery session, all of the trainees are required to write up the surgery that they are responsible for the following day. For example, the second-year resident routinely performs all cystoscopic procedures and writes up the cystoscopic procedure by breaking it into its component parts and including a description of instrumentation. The write-up for cystoscopy includes:

Informed consent
±Regional anesthesia
Position (dorsal lithotomy), preparation, and drape
Select scope: 17F catheter sheath, 70-degree scope (diagnostic)
Prepare scope (assemble, white balance, focus)
Place scope with solution on, distend bladder cavity
Adjust scope (focus, aperture)
Locate trigone, intrauteric ridge, ureters
Locate dome of bladder by identifying air bubble
Survey bladder mucosa
Remove scope

During the imagery session, residents are encouraged to add appropriate hand movements to their description of the surgical procedures (eg, pivoting the cystoscope to visualize the ureters or placement of a clamp to incorporate the uterosacral ligaments) (Fig. 1). All trainees involved with the case are present for the session to ensure that the entire operative team is aware of the steps of a procedure and, before entering the operating room, know their particular responsibilities during the case. After each surgical case, the residents complete a "Global Rating Scale of Operative Performance" for the portion of the case that

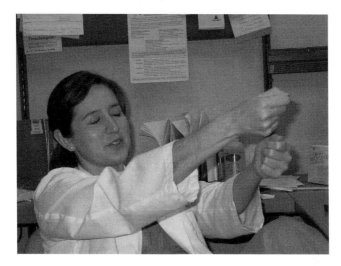

Fig. 1. Resident during mental imagery session.

they perform [19]. The write-ups and Global Rating Scales become part the resident's performance record. Of the 30 residents who have participated in these training sessions, all have ranked the mental imagery sessions as one of the most valuable parts of their training during their 8-week rotation. Many graduated residents report formally incorporating the exercise into their own practice.

References

[1] Driskell JE, Copper C, Moran A. Does mental practice enhance performance? J Appl Psychol 1994;79:481–92.

[2] Batholon S, Dorion D, Darveau S, et al. Cognitive skills analysis, kinesiology, and mental imagery in the acquisition of surgical skills. J Otolaryngol 2005;34:328–32.

[3] Sanders CW, Sadoski M, Bramson R, et al. Comparing the effects of physical practice and mental imagery rehearsal on learning basic surgical skills by medical students. Am J Obstet Gynecol 2004;191:1811–4.

[4] Paivio A. The concept of representation. In: Broadbent DE, McGaugh JL, Mackintosh NJ, et al, editors. Mental representations: a dual coding approach. New York: Oxford University Press; 1986. p. 16–32.

[5] Paivio A. Dual coding theory. In: Broadbent DE, McGaugh JL, Mackintosh NJ, et al, editors. Mental representations: a dual coding approach. New York: Oxford University Press; 1986. p. 53–83.

[6] Ahsen A. The triple code model for imagery and psychophysiology. Journal of Sport and Exercise Psychology 1984;8:15–42.

[7] Martin KA, Moritz SE, Hall CR. Imagery use in sport: a literature review and applied model. The Sport Psychologist 1999;13:245–68.

[8] Vealey RS, Walter SM. Imagery training for performance enhancement and personal development. In: Williams JM, editor. Applied sport psychology: personal growth to peak performance. 2nd edition. Mountain View (CA): Mayfield; 1993. p. 200–24.

 [9] Hall CR, Mack D, Paivio A, et al. Imagery use by athletes: development of the Sport Imagery Questionnaire. Int J Sport Psychol 1998;29:73–89.
[10] Burhans RS, Richman CL, Bergey DB. Mental imagery training: effects on running speed performance. Int J Sport Psychol 1988;19:26–37.
[11] Lee C. Psyching up for a muscular endurance task: effects of image content of performance and mood state. Journal of Sport and Exercise Psychology 1990;12:66–73.
[12] Fenker RM, Lambiotte JG. A performance enhancement program for a college football team: one incredible season. The Sport Psychologist 1987;1:224–36.
[13] Mace RD, Eastman C, Carroll D. The effects of stress inoculation training on gymnastics performance on the pommel horse: a case study. Behavioral Psychotherapy 1987;16:165–75.
[14] MacIntyre T, Moran A, Jennings DJ. Is controllability of imagery related to canoe-slalom performance? Percept Mot Skills 2002;94:1245–50.
[15] Hecker JE, Kaczor LM. Application of imagery theory to sport psychology: some preliminary findings. Journal of Sport and Exercise Psychology 1988;10:363–73.
[16] Liu KP, Chan CC, Lee TM, et al. Mental imagery for promoting relearning for people after stroke: a randomized controlled trial. Arch Phys Med Rehabil 2004;85:1403–8.
[17] Scheuneman AL, Pickleman J, Hesslein R, et al. Neuropsychologic predictors of operative skill among general surgery residents. Surgery 1984;96:288–93.
[18] Gor M, McCloy R, Stone R, et al. Virtual reality laparoscopic simulator for assessment in gynaecology. BJOG 2003;110:181–7.
[19] Reznik R, Regehr G, MacRae H, et al. Testing technical skill via an innovative "bench session" examination. Am J Surg 1997;173:226–30.

**ELSEVIER
SAUNDERS**

Obstet Gynecol Clin N Am
33 (2006) 305–323

OBSTETRICS AND
GYNECOLOGY
CLINICS
OF NORTH AMERICA

Teaching and Evaluating Ultrasound Skill Attainment: Competency-Based Resident Ultrasound Training for AIUM Accreditation

Rebecca Hall, PhD*, Tony Ogburn, MD,
Rebecca G. Rogers, MD

*Department of Obstetrics and Gynecology, University of New Mexico Health Sciences Center,
MSC10 5580, Albuquerque, NM 87131–0001, USA*

Modern obstetrics and gynecology (Ob-Gyn) practice requires the frequent use of ultrasound and ultrasound training as a required component of Ob-Gyn residencies. Although most programs do offer training in obstetric ultrasound imaging, education in gynecologic imaging is either absent or limited. National and international standards in medical imaging require regimented education for physicians in all subspecialty fields of diagnostic ultrasound, including obstetrics and gynecology, genitourinary, vascular, cardiac, gastrointestinal, neurosonology, and others [1–5]. Fellowships in radiology and maternal fetal medicine in diagnostic ultrasound have specific curricula; however, there are no standardized requirements or curricula for residency training in Ob-Gyn.

Ultrasound didactic and clinical education must address the advancing experience and skill levels of each resident [6–9]. A standardized didactic curriculum and ultrasound clinical examination experience may serve the needs of various specialties, including Ob-Gyn and radiology residents and maternal fetal medicine fellows [10]. Specialties other than Ob-Gyn have developed curricula for limited specific skills, such as the focused abdominal sonography for trauma examination, or the focused assessment with sonography for trauma (also known as focused abdominal sonography for trauma). These programs certify non-

---

* Corresponding author.
  E-mail address: rjhall@salud.unm.edu (R. Hall).

0889-8545/06/$ – see front matter © 2006 Elsevier Inc. All rights reserved.
doi:10.1016/j.ogc.2006.02.001

radiologist clinicians in emergency medicine and surgery residencies to rule out blunt abdominal trauma and peritoneal compartment free fluid accumulation. The Family Medicine Advanced Life Support in Obstetrics course includes ultrasound training and has been used to train family medicine residents. Other approaches to residency training in ultrasound have been used by various specialties, including review of still images and assessment of real-time taped examinations as tools for discussion. Other than specifying the number of examinations, however, no specific criteria for standardized competency have been described for Ob-Gyn residents [11–16].

Guidelines for Ob-Gyn and radiology resident ultrasound training have been developed by the American College of Obstetrics and Gynecology, the International Society of Ultrasound in Obstetrics and Gynecology, the Association of Program Directors in Radiology, the American Institute of Ultrasound in Medicine (AIUM), the curriculum committee of the Society of Radiologists in Ultrasound, and the Council on Resident Education in Obstetrics and Gynecology (CREOG) [17–21]. These organizations suggest that trainees have knowledge of multiple medical areas to perform or interpret ultrasound examinations; however, specific components of a structured curriculum are not described [20,22–24]. In addition to the need for standardized education in ultrasound, medical insurers are beginning to require proved competency in sonography, including credentialing of examiners and laboratory accreditation, for reimbursement.

The AIUM accredits ultrasound imaging laboratories. The process for successful accreditation addresses both required credentialing of examiners of the imaging laboratory and qualifications of the interpreting physician. Successful accreditation through the AIUM demonstrates the highest quality of national medical imaging standards for the practicing physician. The University of New Mexico (UNM) has established a curriculum that meets the requirements for AIUM laboratory accreditation eligibility and addresses the broad requirements outlined in the CREOG Educational Objectives Core Curriculum in Obstetrics and Gynecology, 7th edition [21]. Using CREOG objectives, the curriculum sets forth specific requirements to enhance standardization in ultrasound training in Ob-Gyn programs.

This article describes a comprehensive ultrasound curriculum for Ob-Gyn residents that has been developed and implemented at the UNM. The curriculum is competency based and qualifies the graduating resident to seek AIUM laboratory accreditation.

The University of New Mexico curriculum overview

The UNM required curriculum includes dedicated didactic lectures, laboratory imaging case study review, individual daily clinical case discussions, patient care conferences, reading assignments, learning objectives review, two written comprehensive examinations, and completion of multilevel clinical competencies. The authors have developed a model for competency-based skill assessment so that the inconsistent experience that is inherently varied among resident rotations can be systematically approached for each resident with the intention of standardizing skill development. Areas covered include:

Cross-sectional anatomy of the female pelvis
Review of gynecologic imaging, including CT and diagnostic ultrasound
Normal gynecologic ultrasound examination
Translabial assessment of the female urethra and anal sphincter complex
Abnormal gynecologic ultrasound examination
    Additional examination tools to use in the presence of pathology
    Differential diagnosis
    How to follow-up on abnormal examination findings
Sonohydrohysterography
    Performance of the procedure
    Findings of normal uterus and endometrium
    How the procedure enhances confidence of findings associated with
       abnormal uterus and endometrium
First trimester imaging and assessment
    Embryology and prenatal development
    Endovaginal examination
    Nuchal translucency
    Mullerian abnormalities
    First trimester emergency pathologies (ectopic pregnancy, imminent
       abortion, and so forth)
Second and third trimester examination
    AIUM examination protocol
    Biometrics
    Biometric ratios
    Biophysical profile–amniotic fluid index
    Placenta
    Fetal vascularity
    Doppler assessment of the placenta and fetus
    Central nervous system, thoracic, cardiac, gastrointestinal-genitourinary,
       skeletal systems
       Embryology-prenatal development
       Normal examination findings
       Pathologies and associated findings
       Differential diagnosis
Intrauterine growth restriction
Genetic syndromes
Aneuploidy (including trisomies and monosomy)
Pathology case review
Clinical research in ultrasound

Physics and instrumental
   "Knobology" of ultrasound system instrumentation
   Doppler instrumentation
   Bioeffects

This competency-based dedicated 4-year clinical ultrasound educational program is integrated throughout the residency. Each resident completes the

---

Box 1. AIUM requirements for laboratory accreditation

Qualified medical staff will interpret or perform clinical studies in accordance with privileges approved by the physician director of ultrasound. Requirements for all other physicians are as follows:

Must be a physician with a current state license
Must obtain a minimum of 30 hours of Category 1 AMA credits in ultrasound every three years
Must meet the AIUM training Guidelines for Physicians Who Evaluate and Interpret Diagnostic Ultrasound Examinations:
   The training should include methods of documentation and reporting of ultrasound studies. Physicians performing diagnostic ultrasound examinations should meet <u>at least one of the following criteria:</u>
   Completion of an approved residency program, fellowship or post-graduate training, which includes the equivalent of at least three month of diagnostic ultrasound training under the supervision of a qualified physician(s), during which the trainee will have evidence of being involved with the performance, evaluation and interpretation of at least 300 sonograms.
   In the absence of formal fellowship or post-graduate training or residency training, documentation of clinical experience could be acceptable providing the following could be demonstrated
      Evidence of 100 hours of AMA Category I CME activity dedicated to diagnostic ultrasound, and
      Evidence of being involved with the performance, evaluation and interpretation of the images of at least 300 sonograms within a three-year period under the supervision of a qualified physician (s).

From the American Institute of Ultrasound in Medicine; with permission.

---

minimum ultrasound didactic and clinical examination objectives set forth by the AIUM (approved 1997, www.AIUM.org) to be eligible for laboratory accreditation after graduation (Box 1) [25].

Completion of the listed AIUM requirements confirms a competent level of skill for eventual postgraduate practice interpretation and billing for ultrasound examinations. At present, laboratory accreditation is not required for obstetric and gynecologic ultrasound examination billing; however, trends in mandating laboratory accreditation to bill are emerging. Graduates who complete the AIUM prerequisites are eligible to apply for laboratory accreditation.

The University of New Mexico resident didactics

The didactic program consists of a minimum mandatory annual ultrasound lecture series each summer. A series of eight dedicated ultrasound lectures is given in July and August when the department traditionally does not hold Grand Rounds (Box 2). Mandatory attendance of these lectures for 4 years results in 32 hours of sonology lectures, although additional lectures are given individually during clinical rotations and at other department educational meetings. The lectures allow first year residents immediately to begin to attain knowledge in ultrasound and develop advancing clinical applications that they can fine-tune over the 4 years. Twenty additional hours of one-on-one ultrasound case review,

---

Box 2. Schedule for resident summer lecture series

Week 1: Introduction to Ultrasound Imaging; Nomenclature

Week 2: Physical Principles and Instrumentation of Diagnostic Ultrasound; Artifacts and Bioeffects

Week 3: Indirect-Direct Fetal Assessment: Amniotic Fluid Volume Indices, the Biophysical Profile, and Doppler Assessment of the Umbilical Arteries, the Middle Cerebral Arteries and the Ductus Venosus

Week 4: First Trimester Obstetric Examination; What You See When

Week 5: Second and Third Trimester Obstetric Ultrasound Examination

Week 6: Evaluation of the Central Nervous System: Embryology, Prenatal Development, and Imaging

Week 7: Evaluation of the Cardiovascular System: Embryology, Prenatal Development, and Imaging

Week 8: Evaluation of the Gastrointestinal-Genitourinary: Embryology, Prenatal Development, and Imaging

Box 3. Didactic and clinical rotation schedule

HOI

Eight-hour summer lecture series
Obstetric low-risk clinical imaging and assessment
Sixty-four hours supervised ultrasound examination
    performance during an ultrasound rotation
One-on-one clinical case review, instrumentation review,
    and lectures
Competency expectation: completion of beginning first, second,
    and third trimester obstetric category competencies
Comprehensive written and case examination #1

HOII

Eight-hour summer lecture series
Gynecology clinical imaging and assessment
Thirty-two hours supervised ultrasound examination perfor-
    mance during reproductive endocrinology rotation
Competency expectation: completion of beginning gynecology
    category competencies

HOIII

Eight-hour summer lecture series
Genetics and high-risk obstetric examinations and prenatal
    diagnosis and assessment
One hundred twenty eight hours supervised ultrasound
    examination performance
One-on-one clinical case review, instrumentation review,
    and lectures
Competency expectation: completion of intermediate first,
    second, and third trimester category competencies
Comprehensive written and case examination #2

HOIV

Eight-hour summer lecture series
Maternal fetal medicine high-risk imaging assessment and
    clinical correlation
Sixty-four hours minimum in-patient supervised ultrasound
    examination performance

Competency expectation: completion of advanced first, second, and third trimester obstetric category competencies
Emergency imaging and assessment

The total number of supervised clinical ultrasound (at least 300 hours) is distinct from the accumulated ultrasound examination hours experienced by residents who are unsupervised by attending faculty.

formal resident education sessions, and informal lectures are given during clinical rotations.

The University of New Mexico resident clinical rotations

The clinical ultrasound requirement consists of a minimum of 300 hours of directly supervised obstetric and gynecologic ultrasound examinations, including the normal obstetric and high-risk obstetric ultrasound examination, abnormal triple-marker screening, transabdominal and endovaginal gynecologic ultrasound, amniocentesis, and other specialized intraoperative ultrasound-guided procedures. This requirement is met during dedicated rotations each year (Box 3). At the beginning of the clinical ultrasound rotations, each resident is given an educational outline from which to prepare for their rotation and an end of rotation written examination. Completion of the clinical training ensures sufficient skill to detect major abnormalities, perform triage for gynecologic emergencies, and make appropriate referrals to tertiary-care centers for further investigations.

The University of New Mexico resident competency-based assessment

Specific examination subcomponents are applied in manageable advancing increments, including instrumentation and knowledge-based associated assessments to detect normal and pathologic findings. The building of understanding and skill development evolves without overwhelming the resident, whereas small documented successes build confidence at each level.

Individual resident competencies are assessed separately for three categories: (1) first trimester obstetric, (2) second and third trimester obstetric, and (3) gynecologic ultrasound examinations. Each category is assessed at three levels: (1) beginning, (2) intermediate, and (3) advanced. Appendices 1, 2, and 3 represent each of the competency areas being assessed. Each represents a competency card. Each resident has three cards that are filled in over the 4 years, recording their progress.

Box 4. Intern diagnostic ultrasound rotation: study outline for written examination

The purpose of this rotation is to introduce you to proper ultrasound examination techniques in obstetric ultrasound. Be prepared to be clinically tested on the *Beginning Competency Objectives.*

During this rotation, you will be given assigned "Learning Issues," usually every day, which will pertain to patients we may have examined that day or cases we may have discussed. You will be expected to read about those Learning Issues for discussion the next day.

By the end of the rotation, we will have covered some of the common pathologic entities found in Obstetrics and Gynecology (but it will be only a small part of the big picture). Your final examination, which will be the last or second to last day of your rotation, will reflect obstetrics topics we discussed as well as objectives listed below. The goal of the rotation is to make this rotation a satisfying experience with a focused, steep learning curve.

Areas related to diagnostic ultrasound that will be tested, will include the following:

Physics: be able to define the following terms

Gain
Output
Field of view
Time gain compensation curve
Near field
Far field
Focal zone
Artifact
Attenuation
Posterior acoustic enhancement
Reverberation
Posterior acoustic shadow
Dynamic range
Tissue harmonics
Color power Doppler
Color flow Doppler
Doppler spectral waveform
Multi Hertz versus single Hertz transducers (What frequencies do we have on our systems?)

Some instrumentation questions to consider

What is the clinical application difference between [Doppler wave-
   form analysis] and [color Doppler] or [color power Doppler]?
Which one gives a global perspective for vascular flow?
Think of four examples when color flow findings would be
   helpful clinically.
Why should you pick your highest-frequency transducer to
   examine every patient?
As related to spatial resolution, what are the most important
   instrument tools you control?
How does reducing the sector width improve spatial resolution?
How does using a "write" zoom function improve spatial resolution?
What is dynamic range? How is it useful?
What is chroma? How is it useful?

Protocol

There is a difference between "scanning" a patient to take fetal
measurements and "examining" a patient to assess the fetus,
uterus, adnexa, and placenta. You will hopefully move from "picture taking" to more about examination of the fetus throughout
your residency.

What is the absolute protocol for the obstetric ultrasound examination? (Find AIUM and American College of Obstetrics
   and Gynecology protocols)
What is considered when evaluating the fetus beyond the
   suggested protocol?
The bladder is filled for what three reasons for an early transabdominal obstetric or gynecologic ultrasound examination?

Biometric ratios

Understand biometric ratios (these are listed at the end of all
   generated reports). For example, consider the following:
Which ratio would be most abnormal if the fetus has a
   brachycephalic head?
Which ratio would be most abnormal if fetus has severe
   asymmetric intrauterine growth restriction?
What is the clinical utility of abnormal ratios?
How much of a discrepancy occurs for a relationship to be
   "red flagged" by the ultrasound system on the biometric
   ratios?

Bottom line fetal echocardiography

Be able to describe how one obtains a four-chamber cardiac view.
What is being evaluated on the four-chamber view? (Consider size, situs, position, symmetry, and IVS)
What is the most common cardiac anomaly? On which planes would it best be visualized sonographically?

Placenta

Although many laboratories do not grade placentas anymore, this simple act will cause the examiner to evaluate it, rather than ignore it.
What are the grading criteria?
What is normal thickness of the placenta? What should the maximum thickness of the placenta measure at 20 weeks maternal age compared with 30 weeks?
Be able to discuss ''placental lakes.''
What is a better way to describe them?
What are the etiologies for this finding? Which are significant?

Cervix

What are two purposes in checking every cervical os on all obstetric ultrasound examinations?
What is the range of normal cervical length?

Physiology

What does the S/D ratio of the umbilical arteries evaluate? Is this old or current physiologic information?
Should every patient have evaluation of S/D ratio?
What is normal S/D ratio of the umbilical arteries at, for example, 20 weeks versus 36 weeks? What is the mechanism of this difference over time?

Cerebral ventricular system

Normal central nervous system ventricular atrium measurement for ventricles is consistently <10 mm throughout pregnancy.
Give four etiologies that would result in ventriculomegaly (greater than 10 mm).
Why is it important to assess the cerebral mantle in the presence of ventriculomegaly?

Amniotic fluid indices

What maternal conditions are associated with polyhydramnios?
What fetal conditions are associated with polyhydramnios?
A helpful acronym to remember associations for oligohydramnios is DRIPP. Give the etiologies:
D
R
I
P
P

Genitourinary

What are the differences between infantile polycystic kidney disease (autosomal recessive), multicystic dysplastic kidney disease, and adult polycystic kidney disease (autosomal dominant)? Make a chart with the following information completed. Consider etiologies, clinical outcomes, and sonographic findings (echo pattern, unilateral versus bilateral, and size)

Gastrointestinal

Be able to compare gastroschisis versus omphalocele in terms of
Incidence
Etiology
Ultrasound findings
Associated findings
Prognosis

Artistic exercise

Draw a fetus in the cephalic position with the spine on the maternal left.
Draw a line (axial cut) of the fetal abdomen as if you are making a transverse plane ON MOM where you would correctly measure the abdominal circumference (AC).
Draw a separate picture of how that cut would look on the ultrasound plane (where are the correct landmarks on this plane?).
Draw lines at where you would assess the fetal kidneys, posterior fossa, and sagittal spine.

On the card, the horizontal boxes represent individual examinations. The vertical boxes represent each competency within that examination. Every examination performed by the resident addresses all competencies for that particular examination. Individual competencies are informally evaluated, but all must be completed before a resident can attempt to be assessed for an entire examination. Small steps can be confidently obtained before being expected to perform the entire examination on a single patient. Residents complete 10 examinations at the beginning level, and five for both intermediate and advanced levels for each category.

Advancement occurs throughout the 4 years. For example, the intern is expected to complete the beginning competencies for second- and third-trimester obstetric imaging by the end of a 1-month scheduled rotation the first year. The second year resident is expected to complete the beginning competencies for first trimester and gynecology during their 2-month reproductive endocrinology rotation during a weekly gynecology ultrasound clinic. The third year resident is expected to complete the intermediate competencies for the second- and third-trimester obstetric imaging during their genetics–prenatal diagnosis 2-month rotation. Finally, advanced levels of all three areas are to be completed during emergency and maternal fetal medicine rotations by senior level residents. Individual competency cards are kept on file by the program director with expected completion of all competencies by year 4 of residency. Completed cards are placed in the graduating residents' permanent records.

Knowledge-based assessment

Assessment includes both knowledge and competency-based evaluations that are completed during rotations. At the beginning of each rotation, a learning objectives outline is given to each resident (Box 4). In addition to completion of the described competency cards, two written examinations are given that assess knowledge of basic physics and instrumentation, embryology and prenatal development, sonographic findings of the normal and abnormal anatomy, and differential diagnosis of these findings. Testing is conducted at the end of the intern rotation and at the completion of the third year rotation. These examinations include multiple choice questions and "fill in the blank" questions associated with pathologic diagnosis for 30 individual imaging cases.

Summary

Ultrasound examination and interpretation skills are required to practice Ob-Gyn. Resident sonologists must be educated in not only proved competency in the performance, but the interpretation of Ob-Gyn ultrasound examinations.

Adherence to AIUM recommendations confirms quality standards for Ob-Gyn ultrasound examinations. The UNM program requires attendance of 30 lectures throughout residency, and direct supervision of 300 hours of clinical ultrasound examinations to fulfill AIUM requirements for laboratory accreditation. Use of a competency system that is broken down into manageable advancing skill steps standardizes the clinical ultrasound experience and allows for documentation of skill development for all residents. The program at the UNM provides a challenging, yet satisfying experience to accomplish high standards for graduates in Ob-Gyn diagnostic ultrasound imaging.

Appendix 1: Resident ultrasound competency objectives—first trimester obstetric ultrasound examination

Beginning competency level (each objective is a box on the competency form to be checked by evaluator)

1. Choose appropriate transducer per individual patient and procedure.
2. Correctly use instrumentation parameters (time gain compensation, gain, output, focal zone, and so forth).
3. Correctly identify anatomy and plane relationships used for transabdominal ultrasound examination.
4. Recognize uterine and ovarian anatomy in sagittal and transverse planes.
5. Correctly document and measure uterus and ovaries in sagittal, transverse, and anteroposterior diameters.
6. Correctly identify the yolk sac, and extraembryonic mesoderm.
7. Correctly identify, document, and measure the gestational sac.
8. Correctly identify, document, and measure the crown-rump length of the embryo, if present.
9. Describe findings at 5, 6, 7, 8, 9, 10, and 12 weeks' estimated gestational age as related to embryologic development.
10. Know formulas for converting gestational sac and crown rump length to menstrual age.
11. Use proper postexamination clean-up procedures.

Intermediate competency level

1. Correctly perform all beginning competency level criteria as described in the beginning competency level with limited supervision.
2. Correctly examine and document normal adnexa.
3. Correctly document any pathologic findings in the pelvis, including cul de sac fluid or masses in the uterus or adnexa.
4. When transabdominal visualization of embryo is equivocal, be able to perform an endovaginal examination of the pelvis.

5. Correctly assess the embryonic anatomy endovaginally.
6. Correctly use m-mode for fetal heart motion and measure beats per minute.

Advanced competency level

1. Correctly perform all competency level criteria as described in the beginning and intermediate competency levels with limited supervision.
2. Correctly perform color-flow and Doppler waveform analysis of uterine and ovarian arteries.
3. Correctly differentiate between "real" findings and artifacts.
4. Describe a differential diagnosis based on clinical and sonographic findings (to include intrauterine pregnancy, intrauterine pregnancy in a leiomyomatous uterus, decidual reaction to pregnancy, ectopic pregnancy, corpus luteum cysts, presence of cul de sac fluid and adnexal masses).

Resident Ultrasound Competency Objectives

1ST TRIMESTER OBSTETRIC ULTRASOUND EXAM

Resident Name: _____

Beginning	1	2	3	4	5	6	7	8	9	10
1										
2										
3										
4										
5										
6										
7										
8										
9										
10										
11										

Intermediate	1	2	3	4	5
1					
2					
3					
4					
5					
6					

Advanced	1	2	3	4	5
1					
2					
3					
4					

Appendix 2: Resident ultrasound competency objectives—second and third trimester obstetric ultrasound examination

Beginning competency level (each objective is a box on the competency form to be checked by evaluator)

1. Choose appropriate transducer per individual patient and procedure.
2. "Recall" instrumentation settings for appropriate examination parameters.
3. Correctly use standard ultrasound imaging planes in evaluating the pregnant uterus.
4. Correctly identify fetal lie and location of fetal spine and extremities.
5. Be able to describe location and grade of the placenta.
6. Be able to identify cord insert at anterior wall of fetal abdomen and at placenta.
7. Be able to complete individual parameters of obstetric examination protocol with supervision, including:
   Four-chamber heart
   Biparietal diameter
   Femur length, humerus length
   Amniotic fluid volume, both subjectively and by AFI index (after 26 weeks)
   Internal cervical os (transabdominal approach)
   Head circumference
   Abdominal circumference
8. Use proper postexamination clean-up procedures.

Intermediate competency level

1. Perform a complete low-risk obstetric examination by correct documentation of all examination protocol as described at the beginning competency level with limited supervision.
2. Correctly obtain the following additional parameters:
   Ventricular atrium measurement
   Cisterna magnum diameter
   Cervical length
   Cerebellum measurement
   Nuchal cord thickness
3. Perform Doppler systolic and diastolic evaluation of the fetal umbilical artery.
4. Obtain left ventricular outflow tract and right ventricular outflow tract of fetal heart after 20 weeks gestation.

Advanced competency level

1. Perform a complete obstetric ultrasound examination as described at the beginning and intermediate competency levels from the following high-risk categories:
   Multiple gestation
   Congenital anomalies
   Suspected aneuploidy
   Rh isoimmunization
   Gestational diabetes
   High risk for cardiac anomalies
2. Assess the aortic and ductal arches.
3. Identify and correctly document any pathologic findings.
4. Correctly extend examination protocols in the presence of pathology as related to associated findings.
5. Describe differential diagnosis for pathologic findings.

Resident Ultrasound Competency Objectives

2ND & 3RD TRIMESTER OBSTETRIC ULTRASOUND EXAM

Resident Name: _____

Beginning	1	2	3	4	5	6	7	8	9	10
1										
2										
3										
4										
5										
6										
7										
8										

Intermediate	1	2	3	4	5
1					
2					
3					
4					

Advanced	1	2	3	4	5
1					
2					
3					
4					
5					

Appendix 3: Resident ultrasound competency objectives—gynecologic ultrasound examination

Beginning competency level (each objective is a box on the competency form to be checked by evaluator)

1. Choose appropriate transducer per individual patient and procedure.
2. Correctly use instrumentation parameters (TGC, gain, output, focal zone, and so forth).
3. Correctly identify anatomy-plane relationship.
4. Correctly identify bladder, uterus, vagina, ovaries, and posterior cul de sac.
5. Correctly document and measure uterus and ovaries in sagittal and transverse plane.
6. Use proper postexamination clean-up procedures.

Intermediate competency level

1. Correctly perform the gynecologic ultrasound examination as described at the beginning competency level with limited supervision.
2. Correctly document sagittal and transverse images of iliac vessels and pelvic muscles.
3. Correctly evaluate for intraperitoneal fluid collections, particularly the posterior cul de sac and the subhepatic space.
4. Correctly obtain color flow images of uterine and ovarian vasculature.

Advanced competency level

1. Correctly perform the gynecology ultrasound examination as described at the beginning and intermediate competency level with limited supervision.
2. Perform complete endovaginal ultrasound examination.
3. Perform Doppler waveform analysis for resistive index and pulsatility index of ovarian arteries.
4. Correctly differentiate between artifact and "real" findings.
5. Describe a differential diagnosis for pathologic findings.
6. Describe a differential diagnosis for abnormal Doppler resistive indices in the presence of adnexal masses.
7. Perform translabial assessment of the anal sphincter complex.

Resident U/S Competency Objectives

GYN ULTRASOUND EXAM

Resident Name: _____

Beginning	1	2	3	4	5	6	7	8	9	10
1										
2										
3										
4										
5										
6										

Intermediate	1	2	3	4	5
1					
2					
3					
4					

Advanced	1	2	3	4	5
1					
2					
3					
4					
5					
6					
7					

References

[1] Bofill JA, Sharp GH. Obstetric sonography: who to scan, when to scan and by whom. Obstet Gynecol Clin North Am 1998;25:465–78.

[2] Mandavia DP, Aragona J, Chan L, et al. Ultrasound training for emergency physicians: a prospective study. Acad Emerg Med 2000;7:1008–14.

[3] Robinson NA, Clancy MJ. Should UK emergency physicians undertake diagnostic ultrasound examinations? J Accid Emerg Med 1999;16:248–9.

[4] Hofer M, Mey N, Metten J, et al. Quality control of sonography courses in advanced training of physicians: analysis of present status and potential for improvement. Ultraschall Med 2002; 23:89–97.

[5] Heller MB, Bunning ML, France ME, et al. Residency training in emergency ultrasound: fulfilling the mandate. Acad Emerg Med 2002;9:835–9.

[6] American College of Radiology. ACR standards for performing and interpreting diagnostic ultrasound examinations. In: Carroll BA, Babcock DS, Hertzberg BS, et al, editors. Standards. Reston (VA): American College of Radiology; 2000. p. 235–6.

[7] Hertzberg BS, Kliewer MA, Bowie JD, et al. Physician training requirements in sonography: how many cases are needed for competence? AJR Am J Roentgenol 2000;174:1221–7.

[8] Maldjian PD. Physician training requirements in sonography. AJR Am J Roentgenol 2001;176: 1075–6.

[9] Jang T, Sineff S, Naunheim R, et al. Residents should not independently perform focused abdominal sonography for trauma after 10 training examinations. J Ultrasound Med 2004;23: 793–7.

[10] Calhoun BC, Hume Jr RF. Integrated obstetric curriculum for obstetrics and gynecology residency, radiology residency and maternal-fetal medicine fellowship program at an accredited American institute of ultrasound in medicine diagnostic ultrasound center. Ultrasound Obstet Gynecol 2000;16:68–71.

[11] Kirkpatrick AW, Simons RK, Brown R, et al. The hand-held FAST: experience with hand-held trauma sonography in a level-I urban trauma center. Injury 2002;33:303–8.

[12] Kirkpatrick AW, Sirois M, Ball CG, et al. The hand-held ultrasound examination for penetrating abdominal trauma. Am J Surg 2004;187:660–5.

[13] Rozycki GS, Ballard RB, Feliciano DV, et al. Surgeon-performed ultrasound for the assessment of truncal injuries: lessons learned from 1540 patients. Ann Surg 1998;228:557–67.

[14] Sisley AC, Johnson SB, Erickson W, et al. Use of an objective structured clinical examination (OSCE) for the assessment of physician performance in the ultrasound evaluation of trauma. J Trauma 1999;47:627–31.

[15] Nunes LW, Simmons S, Hallowell MJ, et al. Diagnostic performance of trauma US in identifying abdominal or pelvic free fluid and serious abdominal or pelvic injury. Acad Radiol 2001;8: 128–36.

[16] Counselman FL, Sanders A, Slovis CM, et al. The status of bedside ultrasonography training in emergency medicine residency programs. Acad Emerg Med 2003;10:37–42.

[17] International Society of Ultrasound in Obstetrics and Gynecology. Proposed minimum standards for ultrasound training for residents in obstetrics and gynecology. Ultrasound Obstet Gynecol 1993;3:73–6.

[18] Rao VM. ACR standards for performing and interpreting diagnostic ultrasound examinations. Reston, Viginia: American College of Radiology. Revised 2000. Available at: www.apdr.org/programdirector/introduction.htm 2001. Accessed March 7, 2006.

[19] AIUM. Practice accreditation. Available at: http://www.aium.org/accreditation/practice/one.asp. Accessed March 7, 2006.

[20] Townsend R, Frates M, Goldstein R, et al. Ultrasound. Curriculum committee of the Society of Radiologists in Ultrasound. Available at: www.apdr.org/programdirector/ultrasound.htm. Accessed March 7, 2006.

[21] Education Committee of the Council on Resident Education in Obstetrics and Gynecology (CREOG). Educational objectives: core curriculum in obstetrics and gynecology. 7th edition. Washington: Council on Resident Education in Obstetrics and Gynecology; 2002.

[22] World Health Organization Study Group. Training in diagnostic ultrasound: essentials, principles and standards. Technical Report Series. Geneva: World Health Organization; 1998.

[23] Connor PD, Deutchman ME, Habn RG. Training in obstetric sonography in family medicine residency programs: results of a nationwide survey and suggestions for a teaching strategy. J Am Board Fam Pract 1994;7:124–9.

[24] American Society of Diagnostic and Interventional Nephrology. Guidelines for training, certification and accreditation in renal sonography. Semin Dial 2002;15:442–4.

[25] AIUM. Practice accreditation: training guidelines for physicians who evaluate and interpret diagnostic ultrasound examinations. Available at: http://www.aium.org/accreditation/practice/one.asp. Accessed March 7, 2006.

ELSEVIER
SAUNDERS

Obstet Gynecol Clin N Am
33 (2006) 325–332

OBSTETRICS AND
GYNECOLOGY
CLINICS
OF NORTH AMERICA

How to Teach and Evaluate Learners in the Operating Room

Kimberly Kenton, MD, MS

*Division of Female Pelvic Medicine and Reconstructive Surgery, Departments of Obstetrics and
Gynecology and Urology, Loyola University Medical Center, 2160 South First Avenue,
Maywood, IL 60153, USA*

You cannot learn to play the piano by going to concerts.

Increasing financial and medicolegal demands paired with limited resident work hours have forced a change in the apprenticeship model of surgical training. Mounting literature supports a shift to outside of the operating room as the primary site of resident surgical training [1–5]. Several advantages accompany this paradigm shift, which have been addressed elsewhere in this issue. Ultimately, however, surgical competency must be obtained in the operating room. A survey of United States obstetric and gynecology residency program directors assessed how surgical skills are taught and 100% of residency programs reported teaching surgical skills in the operating room [6]. Eighty-eight percent also used lectures, whereas only 68% used bench procedures or models, and 54% practiced procedures on animal models. Only 29% of residency programs had a formal surgical skills curriculum. Furthermore, whereas some cognitive and technical skills can and should be practiced outside the operating room, no laboratory or simulator can ultimately duplicate the operating room experience. Unlike surgical simulators and laboratories, each patient and case is unique and the young surgeon must learn to adapt, problem solve, and retain their composure in real-life circumstance.

Little data exist on actual teaching in the operating room. Most academic surgeons rely on expert opinion and experience for effective teaching and

E-mail address: kkenton@lumc.edu

0889-8545/06/$ – see front matter © 2006 Elsevier Inc. All rights reserved.
doi:10.1016/j.ogc.2006.02.003

evaluation techniques. Attending surgeons and residents do not always agree on which factors are important for teaching in the operating room. A postal survey of 89 attending physicians who were members of the Chicago Gynecologic Society and 38 obstetric and gynecology residents in Chicago identified 10 factors as important for teaching in the operating room, including attending surgeon's knowledge of anatomy, attending surgeon's willingness to teach, ability of attending surgeon to show the resident how to do the case, good exposure, formative feedback, lighting, letting the resident do the case, attending surgeon's patience and calm temperament, and observing a skilled surgeon [7].

Of the listed factors, the top three items valued by the attending surgeons were (1) knowledge of anatomy, (2) exposure, and (3) skill of attending surgeon. In contrast, the top three items ranked by the residents were (1) the attending surgeon's willingness to teach, (2) knowledge of anatomy, and (3) letting the resident do the case. Significantly more residents than attending surgeons rated the following as important: the supervising surgeon's willingness to teach ($P<.0005$); the supervising surgeon's willingness to let the resident do the case ($P<.0005$); and a supervising surgeon with a calm temperament ($P=.03$) and patience ($P=.026$).

Developing into a competent surgeon requires acquisition of both cognitive and motor skills. Spencer [8] proclaimed that 75% of surgical competency is related to decision making, whereas only 25% is related to technical skills. Many aspects of both cognitive and motor skill development can be achieved outside the operating room. Surgical anatomy can be mastered using surgical atlases and cadaveric dissections. Steps of the procedure, instrumentation, and problem solving can be memorized and drilled by the resident alone and in preoperative conferences. Motor skills can be practiced in surgical skill laboratories. Outlines for mastering technical skills include development of both cognitive and motor skills [9–11]. Kopta [9] described one program that lists three steps to develop technical competence: (1) perception, (2) integration, and (3) automatization. First, learners develop a perception or mental image of the task to be performed. The mental image is then integrated with motor or surgical skills with active effort on the part of the learner. Finally, over time, the young surgeon is automatically able to perform each portion of the operation.

Although many aspects of Kopta's [9] program can be taught outside the operating room, certain components must be learned in the operating room. A variety of techniques are used to develop a mental image of the skill to be learned including surgical atlases, cadaveric dissections, and surgical videos. Direct observation of more senior surgeons in the operating room is essential, however, to form an accurate mental image. Direct observation combined with opportunities for surgical practice have been shown to be more beneficial than either alone [12]. Only by seeing visual and spatial relationships, exploring tissue planes and textures, and observing surgeon-assistant interactions during real cases can the trainee fully develop a solid mental image of the skills to be learned.

Cardinal motor skills, including knot tying, suturing, and clamp placement, are probably the easiest surgical skills to learn outside the operating room and can be practiced in skills laboratories. Models and simulators can be used for more complex skills. Essential components, however, such as the way tissues feel when the surgeon is in the correct surgical plane, must be mastered in the operating room. The final step in surgical competency, automatization, also ultimately requires real operating room experience and repetition. The ability to do a case start to finish, adapt to the particulars of that case and patient's anatomy, and direct surgical assistants and other operating room personal all require operating room experience. It is only through experience that one confidently learns to manage all aspects of the surgery competently.

How does one teach once in the operating room? Few attending physicians have formal training in education, and little peer-reviewed literature exists to guide surgical teaching practices. Most academic surgeons accomplish surgical teaching based on their own educational experiences by incorporating what worked when they themselves were trainees and discarding what did not work. With paradigm changes in surgical training programs, methods used in the past, which were based on large volume repetition, may be less effective in ensuring competency than they were in the past.

At Loyola University, several techniques are used to improve teaching in the operating room and patient safety. Expectations are set before each case, so that each member of the team knows for which portion of the procedure they are responsible. All teams function better when everyone clearly understands his or her role. This is true in athletics, business, education, and surgery. When team members (and students) know what to expect, they can mentally and physically prepare for the task ahead. This optimizes everyone's performance and dramatically reduces miscommunication and frustration, which decrease both trainee learning and patient safety. Immediately before the case what each member of the surgical team does is reviewed. For example, the medical student knows he or she places the Foley catheter, the resident opens and closes the abdomen with the fellow, and the fellow performs the sacrocolpopexy. This way, each surgical team member knows what to expect during that case. This facilitates efficiency by cueing team members when to rotate positions at the operating table and identifying who should take charge of which portion of the case (call for instruments, direct assistants, and so forth). It also decreases disappointment and frustration, which can lead to decreased efficiency.

"Forward motion" is the term for efficiency in the operating room, and it is taught actively. Most surgical education programs focus on development of cognitive and technical skills, but fail to teach the practical aspects of intraoperative management. At Loyola University, it is stressed to residents and fellows that they should never be standing around in the operating room. Anesthesia induction time is used just before the case: to position the lights so they are aimed at the appropriate parts of the pelvis or vagina and can be easily adjusted during the case; and to position the patient in dorsal lithotomy and to review proper limb placement in stirrups to avoid neural injuries. Equipment and suture pulled for the procedure is checked before the case begins to avoid unnecessary waiting and delays during surgery.

At Loyola University, an algorithm for surgical struggling was also developed, which all residents and fellows are encouraged to memorize and use (Fig. 1). As most surgical educators have realized, human nature seems to dictate, "if I just keep trying eventually it will work." Many have watched residents try to place a stitch four or five times without adjusting their technique. Knowing that if you did not get it done with the first or second attempt that you are probably not going to get it done the third or fourth without changing something is not intuitive to most trainees. As a result, residents are actively taught to go through the algorithm when they are struggling. Often, the problem the trainee is struggling with falls on the list. Before the resident can run the checklist himself or herself, the attending physician prompts them through the list in the operating room. Then, when the residents are familiar and comfortable with the list, they can

---

STRUGGLING

↓

How is my lighting?
Do I need to readjust the lights?
Do I need a head-lamp?
Would a lighted retractor improve visibility?

↓

How is my exposure?
Is my retraction optimal?
Would a different retractor work better?
Do I need to repack?

↓

How is the table height?
Is the table to high?
Is the table to low?

↓

How are my instruments?
Do I need longer or shorter instruments?
Would a different shaped clamp work better here?
Do I need pick-ups with teeth instead of smooth?

Fig. 1. Algorithm for surgical struggling.

Box 1. Burch urethropexy

Before a gynecology or urology resident is allowed to participate in a Burch urethropexy, he or she must display certain cognitive knowledge, then a series of technical skills. This typically occurs over several conferences and cases.

1. In the weekly preoperative conference, the resident must be able to list indications and alternatives for the procedure, review important anatomy and landmarks, discuss intraoperative and postoperative complications, and dictate the steps of the procedure. If he or she can do this well, he or she is ready to move on to step 2.
2. At the scrub sink just before the first case, the resident again must review the steps of the procedure (suture, instruments, and so forth).
3. First case: The resident is taught to open the retropubic space on their side. They are then asked to identify important anatomic and surgical landmarks (bladder, Cooper's ligament, obturator notch and neurovascular bundle, and arcus tendineus fascia pelvis). If they are able to meet all of these requirements, then they advance on their next case.
4. Second case: The resident again opens the retropubic space and identifies anatomic landmarks, reinforcing what they learned in the first case. The resident is also allowed to pass the suture arms through Cooper's ligament after the primary surgeon places the vaginal stitches. Some residents are not proficient rotating their wrist and using Heaney needle drivers and struggle here. If they cannot do this easily, then they are not ready to place the vaginal sutures on the next case. During postoperative review of the case, most residents who have had difficulty are able to identify it and electively do not move on in the next case. The resident also places his or her hand in the vagina, while the Burch sutures are tied, to begin learning where to place the urethrovesical junction and how tight to tie the sutures.
5. Third case: Once the resident has achieved the technical competence easily to pass sutures through Cooper's ligament, he or she is ready to place the vaginal sutures. First, he or she again opens the retropubic space and identifies landmarks. Then, with their nondominant hand in the vagina, the resident places the vagina stitches.

typically run the checklist and identify the problem in a matter of minutes, which decreases their frustration and improves patient care.

Finally, an ordered set of criteria has been developed for each surgical procedure, which is shared with the residents at the beginning of the rotation. This re-enforces expectations, helps faculty evaluate the resident's cognitive and technical skills in a structured format, and ensures patient safety by not letting a resident advance until they have mastered the basics. Several examples are shown in Boxes 1 and 2.

This clear, stepwise approach to teaching in the operating room has improved the educational experience for residents and fellows, decreased tension in the operating room, and ensured the safety of patients. It also facilitates attending-

---

Box 2. Intraoperative cystoscopy

Residents are taught routinely to perform intraoperative cystoscopy to evaluate the lower urinary tract. Again, they must meet several criteria outside and inside the operating room before doing this portion of the case.

1. Preoperative conference: The cystoscopy is used as a method of reinforcing residents' knowledge and evaluation of lower urinary tract safety during pelvic surgery. During preoperative conference the resident must be able to discuss the indications, risks, benefits, and complications of cystoscopy, and go through the entire intraoperative work-up of lower urinary tract injuries. They also must display knowledge about instrumentation (types of telescopes, degree of lens, and so forth).
2. First case: The resident learns to assemble the cystoscope, choose between a 30- and 70-degree lens for diagnostic and operative cystoscopy, and identify different types of bridges. They then observe a more senior surgeon performing the cystoscopy, while the senior surgeon explains what they are doing.
3. Second case: The resident is asked to select and assemble the appropriate telescope. If they can do this, they are allowed to start the cystoscopy concentrating on finding the dome, trigone, and ureteral orifices. A more senior scans the urothelium and checks for foreign bodies.
4. Third case: The resident again assembles the scope and checks for ureteral patency. When they can do this easily, they are taught to check the entire urothelium for abnormalities or foreign bodies.

resident feedback during and after the case, by having a set-learning objective for the case, which can be focused on and reviewed.

Evaluation and feedback on operative performance are the final components of teaching in the operating room. Evaluation and feedback should be given in several forms (formative during and after the case and summative at the middle or end of the rotation). When teaching motor skills, it is commonly accepted that feedback should be given as close to the actual performance as possible [13]. Some feedback should even be given during the case to aid the resident and protect the patient; however, this type of feedback should be limited in quantity because resident learners can become overloaded. Feedback during the case needs to be nonpersonalized and focused on the skill or action to be changed. It is also helpful to identify if the resident is a visual or verbal learner because this affects what forms of communication work best. The feedback should be concrete. For example, instead of saying, "take a bigger bite, more laterally," which is nonspecific, say "rotate your needle driver 180 degrees, so the needle enters the tissue at a right angle. Then, place your stitch 1.5 cm lateral to the bladder." Frequently, this simple, concrete instruction enables the resident to make the correction. If he or she is still unable to make the correction, they may be a visual learner. Visual learners benefit from observation, so demonstrate exactly what you want them to do. In addition, if you and the resident have mutually agreed on expectations before the case, they are often more responsive and respond less defensively to intraoperative feedback.

Feedback immediately after the case is equally valuable and is the evaluative component most often neglected. After each case, the author conducts a 5- to 10-minute session with the resident to review what went well and areas for improvement. She frequently starts by asking the resident how they think they did. What went well? What could have gone better? What areas did they identify for improvement? Did they meet the objectives agreed on before the case? Typically, the astute resident can identify most areas themselves, which facilitates the discussion and decreases tension. It also teaches them the life-long skill of self-assessment, so they learn to evaluate their performance after each and every case to improve. During this session, the trainee is also encouraged to develop a "practice plan" before the next case. Maybe they need to practice suturing, removing clamps with their nondominant hand, review anatomy or the steps of the procedure. Finally, summative feedback should be given at the completion of the rotation. This summarizes the resident's strengths and identifies area for continued improvement. If appropriate and effective formative feedback was given during the rotation, the summative evaluation should never be a surprise.

Although the operating room remains the most widely used format for teaching surgical skills, the number of hours residents spend in the operating room continues to decrease. In addition to developing other formats for teaching cognitive and technical surgical skills, there is a need to maximize the time spent in the operating room. Several teaching and evaluation techniques that the author found useful have been reviewed. Little scientific data exist as a guide, however, emphasizing the need for high-quality multicenter educational research.

References

[1] DaRosa DA, Bell RH. Graduate surgical education redesign: reflections on curriculum theory and practice. Surgery 2004;136:966–74.

[2] Goff B, Mandel L, Lentz G, et al. Assessment of resident surgical skills: is testing feasible? Am J Obstet Gynecol 2005;192:1331–8.

[3] Goff BA, Lentz GM, Lee D, et al. Development of a bench station objective structured assessment of technical skills. Obstet Gynecol 2001;98:412–6.

[4] Goff BA, Lentz GM, Lee D, et al. Development of an objective structured assessment of technical skills for obstetric and gynecology residents. Obstet Gynecol 2000;96:146–50.

[5] Goff BA, Nielsen PE, Lentz GM, et al. Surgical skills assessment: a blinded examination of obstetrics and gynecology residents. Am J Obstet Gynecol 2002;186:613–7.

[6] Mandel LP, Lentz GM, Goff BA. Teaching and evaluating surgical skills. Obstet Gynecol 2000;95:783–5.

[7] Kenton K, Fenner D. Survey on teaching in the operating room. Presented at the Society of Gynecologic Surgeons' Annual Meeting. New Orleans, February 28–March 1, 2000.

[8] Spencer C. Teaching and measuring surgical techniques: the technical evaluation of competence. Bull Am Coll Surg 1978;63:9–12.

[9] Kopta JA. An approach to the evaluation of operative skills. Surgery 1971;70:297–303.

[10] Lippert FG, Spolek GA, Kirkpatrick GS, et al. A psychomotor skills course for orthopaedic residents. J Med Educ 1975;50:982–3.

[11] Collins A, Brown JS, Newman SE. Cognitive apprenticeship: teaching the art of reading, writing, and mathematics. In: Resnick LB, editor. Cognition and instruction: issues and agendas. Hillsdale (NJ): Lawrence Earlbaum; 1990. p. 1–34.

[12] Shea CWD, Whitacre C. Actual and observational practice: unique perspective on learning. Res Q Exerc Sport 1993;67:A-79.

[13] Gagne R. The conditions of learning and theory of instruction. 4th edition. New York: Holt, Rinehart and Winston; 1985.

ELSEVIER
SAUNDERS

Obstet Gynecol Clin N Am
33 (2006) 333–342

OBSTETRICS AND
GYNECOLOGY
CLINICS
OF NORTH AMERICA

Avoiding Pitfalls: Lessons in Surgical Teaching

Dee E. Fenner, MD

*Department of Obstetrics and Gynecology, University of Michigan Hospital,
1500 East Medical Center Drive, L4000 Women's Hospital, Ann Arbor, MI 48109–0999, USA*

Surgical mentors play an important role in the educational development of medical students, residents, and fellows. Much of what I have learned about performing and teaching surgery I owe to my own surgical mentors. Since completing my own training, I have become a medical educator, and specifically a teacher of gynecologic surgery. For the past 15 years, I have been a director of residencies and medical student clerkships at two universities. I have also been, and continue to be, an active surgical mentor and teacher of urogynecology fellows. In this article I share lessons I have learned from teaching surgical skills both in and out of the operating room and answer questions that are most commonly asked of me about teaching surgical skills.

Learning surgical skills

Surgical competence entails a combination of knowledge; technical skills; decision making (before, during, and after the operation); communication skills; and leadership skills [1]. Outcome depends not only on the competency of the surgeon but on his or her ability to lead and coordinate a team of skilled personnel including anesthesiologists, nurses, technicians, and surgical assistants (Fig. 1). Acquisition and refinement of basic technical skills by the resident are central and begin the learning process to attain surgical competence. Although much of the knowledge, decision-making skills, and experience needed to become a surgeon must be learned inside the operating room, basic technical skills should be taught and evaluated in the surgical laboratory, outside the operating room. Not all surgeons reach the "top tier" or have the ability to design

E-mail address: deef@med.umich.edu

doi:10.1016/j.ogc.2006.02.005
obgyn.theclinics.com

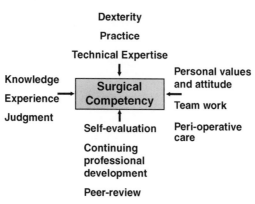

Fig. 1. Surgical competency.

or discover new surgical techniques, but all surgeons must reach an acceptable level of competency (Fig. 2).

Teaching surgical skills in the surgical laboratory

The use of models for laboratory teaching and testing ensures standardization of instruction, feedback, and evaluation. Techniques used to teach and evaluate surgical skills are derived from experience gained from other disciplines that require technical skills assessment, such as flying an airplane. Many learning theories describe the acquisition of surgical skills and other tasks. The behaviorists describes three phases: (1) the cognitive phase or the learning of steps or basic skills, (2) the associative phase where steps learned become part of procedure, and (3) the autonomous phase where the skills can be executed smoothly without any cognitive input. All technical skills can be assessed, from tying a square knot to performing an abdominal hysterectomy. The initial step in teaching

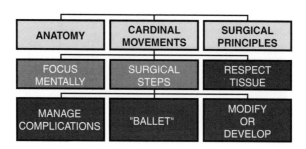

Fig. 2. Basic surgical skills and principles should be learned in a laboratory setting as illustrated in the top row. Learning to focus mentally and putting the surgical steps together begins in the laboratory and continues in the operating room. Higher level skills, such as managing complications, come with experience.

long ago stopped thinking about how to tie a square knot or the steps and motions that his or her hands do to perform this task. He or she is unconsciously competent in this skill. Senior medical students or intern physicians still need to think about the motions involved in tying including how to grasp the suture or cross his or her hands to tie a square knot. He or she is consciously competent. When the teacher is one level above the learner, basic skills can be taught with less effort. The expert, however, must still be sure that all of the steps have been clearly defined and adhered to during teaching. One level above is best for teaching basic skills, but for evaluation, the expert is best for grading.

Teaching in the operating room

When most educators think of a curriculum, they think of a course or series of lectures or laboratories conducted over time. When teaching in the operating room the same basic concepts apply: know your learner, have a set of objectives and ways to teach those objectives in mind, and provide feedback (Fig. 4).

To provide effective feedback the attending physician must be aware of the experience of the trainee. In many cases it is difficult to know how many procedures a particular resident has done. They rotate to other hospitals, scrub with different attendings, and perform an ever increasing variety of procedures. With more residency programs rotating residents to several hospitals, more academic faculty and attending physicians, and fewer gynecologic surgeries being performed nationally, the luxury of working closely with one or two surgical mentors is rare. A resident often scrubs with a different attending every few cases or rotates to a nonsurgical block for several weeks or months. As the attending physician, it is challenging to help the resident build on mistakes or improve surgical skills when one does not know how well the resident performed last week or what are the resident's deficiencies.

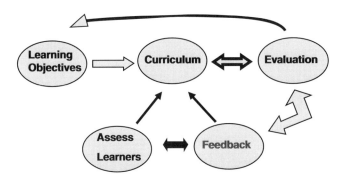

Fig. 4. Curriculum design. The model can be used to design a single teaching opportunity in the operating room. Know the learner, set objectives, assess and provide feedback, and adjust objectives based on performance.

Communication before a case begins can help alleviate some of this problem. To keep within the educational framework as the attending one must assess the learner's level of expertise. For instance, if it is the first time a resident has done a laparoscopic tubal ligation your objectives, mode of instruction, "curriculum," or objectives that you need to teach are different than if it is the tenth or eleventh laparoscopic tubal ligation he or she has performed. For example, ask the resident, "How many vaginal hysterectomies have you performed? For you, what is the hardest part of the procedure to do? What are your weaknesses? What do you want to learn today?." Set that task as the objective for the day and build on the resident's skills.

As a faculty surgeon, it is your obligation to know what skills and procedures a resident is expected to know during each year of training. Your residency program should have a defined set of surgical skills or procedures by resident year of training that can be your guide. These objectives are required by the Residency Review Committee. Most programs use the Council on Residency Education of Obstetrics and Gynecology Objectives as a model. The American Urogynecologic Society also has a set of learning objectives for residents and the Association of Professors of Obstetrics and Gynecology has objectives including procedures for medical students.

For many reasons, such as time restraints, patient safety, and resident education, it is difficult actively to involve medical students in surgical learning. Keep in mind that students do not necessarily have to be actually performing a procedure to be involved. There are several ideas listed that seem to work for me to keep the medical students actively learning while in the operating room.

1. As the attending, talk and teach from the beginning of the procedure until the end. Explain to the resident and student exactly what you are doing and why you are doing that part of the procedure in a certain way. Why you hold a certain clamp and place it the way you do, why you cut the pedicle this way, or why and how you identify the ureter. If a senior resident is the primary surgeon have him or her use the same technique to describe what they are doing to the student. It is a great way to test the resident's knowledge at the same time.
2. Ask only pertinent anatomic questions. Have clear learning objectives in mind that are important for the student to know.
3. Be sure the student can see the operative field at all times. If they cannot, do not make them stand there, scrubbed and bored. If they are only observing, have the student scrub out and find a position where they can see.
4. If the student cannot tie a knot or has never sutured set up a folded blue towel on the corner of the scrub nurse's table. Give the student an extra needle holder, forceps, and suture and let them practice sewing the towel. You can watch them out of the corner of your eye and give them feedback. In only takes a few seconds to check their knots. Then, when the opportunity arises, they are prepared actively to participate.

5. Let the student open the uterus on benign cases once the specimen is out. We routinely bivalve the uterus to check for uterine pathology. Let the student do this on a back table. If everything looks fine they can even try placing a stitch and closing the uterus for more experience with real tissue.

Another difficult and anxiety-provoking situation in the operating room is when two residents or a resident and fellow are scrubbing on the same case. Which resident is going to do what? What is the role of the medical student? These questions should be answered before entering the operating room. Every member of the surgical team should know his or her learning objective for the case and what his or her role is during the surgery, before entering the operating room.

Several years ago an expert panel of surgical educators, including Richard Resnick from the University of Toronto and Ray Lee from the Mayo Clinic, spoke at a break-out session at the Association of Professors of Obstetrics and Gynecology–Council on Residency Education of Obstetrics and Gynecology Objectives annual meeting. When asked what they thought was the most important controllable factor that impacts learning in the operating room, both responded stress. Excess stress in the operating room stops teaching in its tracks. Having an even temper, leading the surgical team, and keeping egos out the operating room keep stress at a minimum. At the same time, high expectations, directing the surgical team to focus on the surgery and patient, and careful attention to details enhances learning. The master surgical educator finds the right balance between extrinsic pressures that encourage learning and the negative effects of being too critical and demanding. When surgical students are intimidated they cannot learn or perform. A modified diagram from Whitman [3] illustrates the relationship between stress and learning (Fig. 5).

Teaching in the operating room requires constant communication between the teacher and student. The senior surgeon should be demonstrating, instructing, or providing feedback at all times. Skills, such as correct positioning of the clamp, proper hand rotation, and conserving motion, should be reinforced and

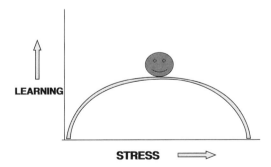

Fig. 5. Stress and learning. As stress increases, learning increases to a point, but as tension and pressure continue to rise, learning declines.

demanded for each step of the procedure. The senior surgeon must not be lazy or distracted, but focused on perfect surgical performance.

Evaluating surgical skills

Evaluation of any skill is a summation of past performance. As seen in the model of curricular design, feedback and evaluation are linked. An evaluation should never be a surprise if feedback has been given during a course, a surgical laboratory session, or in the operating room.

Mandel and coworkers [4] surveyed 266 residency programs in the United States in 1999 concerning their methods used for teaching and evaluating surgical skills. Two hundred twenty-three programs responded to the mailing (76% response rate). Thirty percent of the programs reported formalized curriculum for teaching surgical skills. Overall, only 74% of programs evaluated surgical skills, with over half using subjective faculty evaluations known to have poor reliability and unknown validity. It was these types of studies, increasing concerns for patient safety, and the hope of inspiring life-long learners, which led the Accreditation Council for Graduate Medical Education (ACGME) to develop the Outcomes Project.

The Outcomes Project and Accreditation Council for Graduate Medical Education competencies

In September of 1997, the ACGME endorsed a shift in the focus of residency accreditation from structure and process to educational outcomes. The old structure determined only whether a program had the potential to educate residents, whereas the outcome model determines whether residents are actually being educated. The ultimate goal from the ACGME perspective is to improve the quality of graduate medical education and thereby to enhance the quality of medical care. Unlike before, the shift in education and documentation has gone from lists of learning objectives, lectures, and learning opportunities to documentation that the residents have actually met standardized requirements and achieved a level of competency. "Competency" has become the new paradigm of medical education and certification.

To provide valid surgical evaluations, Reznick and his colleagues at the University of Toronto developed and tested the use of Objective Structured Assessment of Technical Skills (OSATS) [5]. Borrowing from the previously described cognitive task analysis for teaching surgical skills, the process requires establishing set criteria against which technical skills can be assessed. The criteria clearly define how a task should be performed with descriptions of what is correct and what is wrong. Reznick's global ratings scale has been adapted and recommended for use by the ACGME and can be found on their website at www.ACGME.org under the heading "Toolbox."

In a series of educational experiments, Reznick and the team at the University of Toronto [6–8] found that the OSATS system had excellent interrater reliability; that novices scored lower than the senior residents (construct validity); that realistic models worked as well as live animals for teaching technique; and that the system and methods were transferable to other institutions. Similar work at the University of Washington has confirmed the same outcomes for obstetrics and gynecology residents using specialty-specific OSATS. In addition, these researchers proved that by using standardized assessment forms, evaluators could assess their own residents as reliably as someone who did not know the residents [9–11].

Exactly how many evaluations are needed reliably to assess a resident's skills is not known. Currently, residency programs use global rating and assessment forms in different ways. Some require all surgeries to be graded using the global rating scale, a procedure-specific scale, or both. Other programs only evaluate the resident at the end of a rotation or when the resident believes that he or she is "competent" in a certain procedure and asks the attending to do an evaluation as a "pass or fail" for that procedure.

Fung Kee Fung and colleagues [12] at the University of Ottawa used an interactive voice response system to assess residents' laparoscopic skills. Senior residents and faculty graded residents using a 5-point Likert scale. Three ratings for each surgery were obtained. Thirteen faculty preceptors rated 993 procedures performed by 29 residents and determined that a minimum of 12 preceptor ratings ($G = 0.80$) were needed to obtain reliable measures of residents' surgical skills.

Assessing surgical competency requires more than simply evaluating surgical skills. One must observe behavior, judgment, demeanor, decision making, confidence, and other leadership traits. In my experience, poor performance in the operating room can have a variety of causes, including a knowledge deficit, lack of skill, or a poor attitude. Lack of self-awareness or the inability to assess one's skills is common among novice surgeons. The more novice the learner, the more poorly they self-assess. Additionally, female surgical students tend to underestimate their performance more often than male students.

Clear objectives and direct questions can steer learners toward accurate self assessment. Simply asking, "How do you think you did on that hysterectomy?" can start the process. More specific questions, such as, "How do you think you did identifying the ureter?," focus and direct the learner to particular skill areas that may need improvement. For many learners self assessment or admitting deficits in knowledge or skills does not come easily. Most physicians and surgeons fear not being the "best." Without self-assessment and reflection on one's operative performance, however, the novice (or even the experienced) surgeon cannot learn from mistakes and will not advance as a surgeon.

Summary

Becoming a good surgical educator takes time, patience, and dedication. Providing effective feedback is essential to improving the mentee's surgical skills. The operating room is a costly, high-risk classroom. At best, an obstetrics and gynecology resident has 1000 hours of operating room time to learn to be a competent surgeon. If 100 of these precious hours are spent learning how to tie knots and use a needle driver, it reduces the time available to hone or expand surgical skills or gain competency. Residents must come to the operating room prepared. Using a surgical skills laboratory can help in that preparation but is only effective when feedback is given regarding performance. While in the operating room, the attending physician must constantly direct, critique, and actively teach.

References

[1] Moorthy K, Munz Y, Sarker S, et al. Objective assessment of technical skills in surgery. BMJ 2003;327:1032–7.
[2] Velmahos GC, Toutouzas KG, Sillin LF, et al. Cognitive task analysis for teaching technical skills in an inanimate surgical skills laboratory. Am J Surg 2004;187:114–9.
[3] Whitman N. Essential hyperteaching: supervising medical students and residents. Department of Family Medicine, University of Utah School of Medicine, Salt Lake City, Utah; 1997.
[4] Mandel LP, Lentz GM, Goff BA. Teaching and evaluating surgical skills. Obstet Gynecol 2000;95:783–5.
[5] Martin JA, Regehr G, Reznick RK, et al. Objective Structured Assessment of Technical Skill (OSATS) for surgical residents. Br J Surg 1997;84:273–8.
[6] Winckel CP, Reznick RK, Cohen R, et al. Reliability and construct validity of a structured technical skills assessment form. Am J Surg 1994;167:423–7.
[7] Reznick RK, Regehr G, MacRae H, et al. Testing technical skill via an innovative bench station examination. Am J Surg 1996;172:226–30.
[8] Ault G, Reznick RK, MacRae H, et al. Exporting a technical skills evaluation technology to other sites. Am J Surg 2001;182:254–6.
[9] Goff BA, Lentz GM, Lee DM, et al. Development of an objective structured assessment of technical skills for obstetric and gynecology residents. Obstet Gynecol 1996;96:146–50.
[10] Lentz GM, Mandel LS, Lee DM, et al. Testing surgical skills of obstetric and gynecologic residents in a bench laboratory setting: validity and reliability. Am J Obstet Gynecol 2001;184:1462–70.
[11] Goff BA, Nielson PE, Lentz GM, et al. Surgical skills assessment: a blinded examination of obstetrics and gynecology residents. Am J Obstet Gynecol 2002;186:613–7.
[12] Fung Kee Fung K. Interactive voice response to assess residents' laparoscopic skills: an instrument validation study. Am J Obstet Gynecol 2003;189:674–8.

ELSEVIER
SAUNDERS

Obstet Gynecol Clin N Am
33 (2006) 343–345

OBSTETRICS AND
GYNECOLOGY
CLINICS
OF NORTH AMERICA

Index

Note: Page numbers of article titles are in **boldface** type.

A

Animal models, in surgical education, 253, 261, 263, 284

B

Beef tongue–turkey leg episiotomy repair model, in surgical education, 276–277

Bench models, in surgical education, 261, 263

Box trainers, in surgical education, 285–286, 291, 293

C

Cadaver models, in surgical education, 253, 284

Cognitive task analysis, in surgical education, 336–337

Colpocleisis model, in surgical education, 274–275

D

Dexterity analysis systems, in surgical education, 263–264

E

Ethics, in surgical education, 240–243
  desire to perform new procedures and, 240–242
  industry-sponsored crash courses and, 241–242
  postgraduate monitoring and, 242
  residency program and, 240

F

Fajita–candy bar episiotomy model, in surgical education, 278–279

Female clay pelvis model, in surgical education, 273

G

Global Rating Scale of Operative Performance, in surgical education, 261

I

Imagery, in mental practice, in surgical education, 298–302

Inanimate surgical models.
  See Surgical models.

M

McGill Inanimate System for Training and Evaluation of Laparoscopic Skills program, in surgical education, 285–286

Mental practice, in surgical education, **297–304**
  dual coding approach to, 298
  imagery in, 298–302
  predictors of surgical skills and, 300–301
  University of New Mexico experience with, 302–303

Minimally invasive surgical trainer–virtual reality system, in surgical education, 287, 289

O

Objective Structured Assessment of Technical Skills, in surgical education, 254–256, **259–265,** 340–341
  animal versus bench models in, 261, 263
  bench setting evaluation in, 261
  dexterity analysis systems in, 263–264
  Global Rating Scale of Operative Performance and, 261
  rationale for, 260

0889-8545/06/$ – see front matter © 2006 Elsevier Inc. All rights reserved.
doi:10.1016/S0889-8545(06)00037-4
obgyn.theclinics.com

Operating room experience, in surgical
    education, 254, **325–332**
    attending surgeon versus resident values
        in, 326
    cognitive and motor skills in, 326–327
    evaluation and feedback in, 331
    forward motion in, 327
    sample criteria for, 329, 330
    surgical struggling and, 328–329
    surgical team expectations and, 327

P

Papier-mâché cystoscopy model, in surgical
    education, 277–278

S

Sacrocolpopexy model, in surgical
    education, 274

Sacrospinous ligament fixation model,
    in surgical education, 275–276

Simulators, in surgical education.
    See Virtual reality.

Skills training, in surgical education,
    247–258
    curriculum in, 249–257
        animal versus cadaver models
            in, 253
        components of, 249–250
        educational goals in, 251–252
        effectiveness of, 253–254
        enduring benefits of, 254
        evaluation strategies for, 254–255
        implementation plan for, 255–257
        instructional strategies in, 252–254
        instructional time in, 252
        mechanism for revision of, 256
        needs assessment in, 250
        operating room experience in, 254
        pitfalls of, 257
        rationale statement for, 250, 251
        surgical videos in, 253
        terminal learning objectives in, 252
        virtual reality in, 253
    developing program for, 248–249
    need to change, 247–248

Surgical education
    ACGME outcomes model for, 238
    apprentice model for, 235–236
        need to change, 236
    beyond apprentice model, **233–236**
        goals of, 233–234
        reliability of, 234–235
        validity of, 234

current environment in, 238–239
    decreasing number and variety of
        procedures, 239
    less faculty time for resident
        education, 239
    subjective experience of
        mentor, 239
ethics in. *See* ethics.
in ultrasound skills. *See*
    Ultrasound skills.
mental practice in. *See* Mental practice.
need to change, **237–246**
Objective Structured Assessment of
    Technical Skills in. *See* Objective
    Structured Assessment of
    Technical Skills.
operating room experience in. *See*
    Operating room experience.
pitfalls in, **333–342**
    evaluating surgical skills, 340
    learning surgical skills, 333–334
    teaching in operating room,
        337–340
    teaching in surgical laboratory,
        334–337
        assessing learner's level of
            expertise, 338
        cognitive task analysis in,
            336–337
        communication and,
            339–340
        defining surgical skills, 338
        feedback in, 335–336
        keeping students actively
            learning, 338–339
        stress and, 339
skills training program in. *See*
    Skills training.
surgical curriculum in, 243–245
    funding programs to study teaching
        methods, 245
    teaching models for new
        devices, 245
    time in training and, 244–245
surgical models in. *See* Surgical models.
virtual reality in. *See* Virtual reality.

Surgical models, in surgical education,
    267–281
    animal models, 253, 261, 263, 284
    beef tongue–turkey leg episiotomy repair
        model, 276–277
    cadaver models, 253, 284
    colpocleisis model, 274–275
    development of, technical challenges to,
        271–272
    fajita–candy bar episiotomy repair
        model, 278–279
    female clay pelvis model, 273
    future trends in, 280

inanimate models, 268–271
  advantages of, 269–270
  disadvantages of, 269
  to track trainee performance,
    270–271
McGill Inanimate System for Training
  and Evaluation of Laparoscopic
  Skills program, 285–286
papier-mâché cystoscopy model,
  277–278
sacrocolpopexy model, 274
sacrospinous ligament fixation model,
  275–276
watermelon cesarean delivery model,
  279–280

gastrointestinal system, 315
genitourinary system, 315
instrumentation, 313
physics, 312
physiology, 314
placenta, 314
protocol, 313
University of New Mexico curriculum
  for, 306–309
University of New Mexico resident
  clinical rotations in, 311
University of New Mexico resident
  competency-based assessment in,
  311, 316
University of New Mexico resident
  didactics in, 309–311

U

Ultrasound skills, surgical education in,
  305–323
  AIUM requirements for laboratory
    accreditation in, 308
  competency objectives in—first
    trimester, 317
  competency objectives in—gynecologic
    examination, 321
  competency objectives in—second and
    third trimesters, 319–320
  didactic and clinical rotation schedule in,
    310–311
  knowledge-based assessment in, 316
  resident summer lecture series in, 309
  study outline for written examination,
    312–315
    amniotic fluid indices, 315
    artistic exercises, 315
    biometric ratios, 313
    cerebral ventricular system, 314
    cervix, 314
    fetal echocardiography, 314

V

Videos, surgical, in surgical skills training, 253

Virtual reality, in surgical education, 253,
  283–296
  assessing surgical skills in, 293–294
  box trainers in, 285–286, 291, 293
  cadaver versus animal models in, 284
  choice of simulators in, 292–293
  costs of, 291–292
  future trends in, 294
  goals of, 285
  McGill Inanimate System for Training
    and Evaluation of Laparoscopic
    Skills program in, 285–286
  minimally invasive surgical trainer–
    virtual reality system in, 287, 289

W

Watermelon cesarean delivery model, in surgical education, 279–280

Changing Your Address?

Make sure your subscription changes too! When you notify us of your new address, you can help make our job easier by including an exact copy of your Clinics label number with your old address (see illustration below.) This number identifies you to our computer system and will speed the processing of your address change. Please be sure this label number accompanies your old address and your corrected address—you can send an old Clinics label with your number on it or just copy it exactly and send it to the address listed below.

We appreciate your help in our attempt to give you continuous coverage. Thank you.

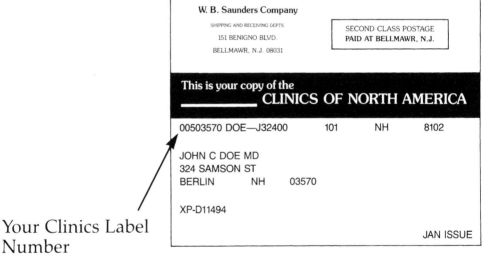

W. B. Saunders Company

SHIPPING AND RECEIVING DEPTS.
151 BENIGNO BLVD.
BELLMAWR, N.J. 08031

SECOND CLASS POSTAGE
PAID AT BELLMAWR, N.J.

This is your copy of the
_____ **CLINICS OF NORTH AMERICA**

00503570 DOE—J32400   101   NH   8102

JOHN C DOE MD
324 SAMSON ST
BERLIN   NH   03570

XP-D11494

JAN ISSUE

Your Clinics Label Number
Copy it exactly or send your label along with your address to:
W.B. Saunders Company, Customer Service
Orlando, FL 32887-4800
Call Toll Free 1-800-654-2452

Please allow four to six weeks for delivery of new subscriptions and for processing address changes.